JOINT DISEASE:
All the arthropathies

E. C. HUSKISSON
Senior Lecturer and Consultant Physician
The Royal Hospital of Saint Bartholomew, London
St. Leonard's Hospital, London

F. DUDLEY HART
Consultant Physician and Rheumatologist
Westminster Hospital, London

Third Edition

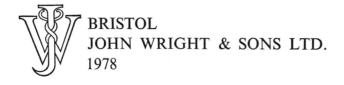

BRISTOL
JOHN WRIGHT & SONS LTD.
1978

CIP Data

Huskisson, Edward Cameron
Joint disease. – 3rd ed
1. Joints – Diseases
I. Title
II. Hart, Francis Dudley
616.7'2   RC932

ISBN 0 7236 0465 7

Printed and bound in Great Britain by REDWOOD BURN LIMITED, Trowbridge & Esher.

CLASSIFICATION OF THE ARTHROPATHIES

INFECTIVE

Infections due to Bacteria, Spirochaetes, and Mycoplasma
Anaerobic infections (p. 6)
Brucellosis (p. 14)
Cat-scratch fever (p. 17)
Clutton's joints (p. 20)
Glanders (p. 38)
Gonococcal arthritis (p. 38)
Infective endocarditis (p. 57)
Leprosy (p. 65)
Melioidosis (p. 72)
Meningococcal arthritis (p. 73)
Mycoplasma arthritis (p. 81)
Rat-bite fever (p. 109)
Salmonella arthritis (p. 118)
Septic arthritis (p. 123)
Septic focus syndrome (p. 124)
Syphilis (p. 130)
Tuberculosis (p. 143)
Typhoid fever (p. 144)
Weil's disease (p. 146)
Yaws (p. 152)

Infections due to Viruses
Adenovirus (p. 3)
Chikungunya (p. 17)
Dengue (p. 24)
Epidemic Australian polyarthritis (p. 29)
Herpes zoster (p. 48)
Lymphogranuloma venereum (p. 70)
Mumps (p. 80)
O'nyong-nyong (p. 17)
Poliomyelitis (p. 99)
Rubella (p. 117)
Smallpox (p. 127)
Vaccination (p. 144)
Varicella (p. 145)
Viral hepatitis (p. 145)

Probably due to Viruses
Erythema infectiosum (p. 30)
Lyme arthritis (p. 69)

Amoebiasis (p. 4)

Infections due to Worms
Acanthocheilonema perstans (p. 1)
Chylous arthritis (p. 19)
Guinea-worm arthritis (p. 40)
Onchocerciasis (p. 87)

Infections due to Fungi
Actinomycosis (p. 36)
African histoplasmosis (p. 3)
Aspergillosis (p. 35)
Blastomycosis (p. 13)
Coccidioidomycosis (p. 21)
Cryptococcosis (p. 35)
Histoplasmosis (p. 49)

Mycetoma (p. 35)
Sporotrichosis (p. 35)

Plant Thorn Synovitis (p. 98)

POST-INFECTIVE
Bacillary dysentery (p. 11)
Henoch-Schönlein purpura (p. 44)
Jaccoud's syndrome (p. 60)
Osteitis pubis (p. 88)
Post-salmonella arthritis (p. 103)
Reiter's disease (p. 110)
Rheumatic fever (p. 113)
Scarlet fever (p. 120)
Yersinia arthritis (p. 152)

METABOLIC AND CRYSTAL DEPOSITION DISEASE
Acid mucopolysaccharidosis (p. 150)
Acute calcific periarthritis (p. 15)
Agammaglobulinaemia (p. 4)
Amyloidosis (p. 5)
Chondrocalcinosis articularis (p. 17)
Dysproteinaemic arthropathy (p. 27)
Familial histiocytic dermatoarthritis (p. 32)
Farber's disease (p. 33)
Gaucher's disease (p. 37)
Gout (p. 39)
Haemochromatosis (p. 41)
Type 2 Hyperlipoproteinaemia (p. 50)
Type 4 Hyperlipoproteinaemia (p. 51)
Hypophosphataemic spondylopathy (p. 55)
Intervertebral disc calcification in children (p. 59)
Morquio-Brailsford syndrome (p. 76)
Mucopolysaccharidoses (p. 78)
Multicentric reticulohistiocytosis (p. 79)
Ochronosis (p. 86)
Osteoarthritis (p. 89)
Pyrophosphate arthropathy (p. 108)
Tumoral calcinosis (p. 144)
Wilson's disease (p. 149)

MECHANICAL AND TRAUMATIC
Gamekeeper's thumb (p. 36)
Genu amoris (p. 37)
Hoffa's disease (p. 50)
Hypermobility syndromes (p. 52)
Instability of the pubic symphysis (p. 58)
Long-leg arthropathy (p. 69)
Occupational arthropathies (p. 85)
Sacro-iliac strain (p. 118)
Temporomandibular pain-dysfunction syndrome (p. 136)
Tennis leg (p. 137)
Traumatic arthritis (p. 142)

CLASSIFICATION OF THE ARTHROPATHIES

The 'Rheumatic' Diseases
Ankylosing spondylitis (p. 7)
Juvenile chronic arthritis (p. 61)
Mixed connective-tissue disease (p. 75)
Palindromic rheumatism (p. 94)
Polyarteritis nodosa (p. 100)
Polymyalgia rheumatica (p. 101)
Polymyositis and dermatomyositis (p. 102)
Rheumatoid arthritis (p. 114)
Scleroderma (p. 121)
Systemic lupus erythematosus (p. 132)

Idiopathic
Acro-osteolysis (p. 2)
Ankylosing vertebral hyperostosis (p. 8)
Arthrogryposis multiplex congenita (p. 9)
Behçet's syndrome (p. 12)
Eosinophilic fasciitis (p. 29)
Familial arthropathy with rash, uveitis and mental retardation (p. 31)
Familial Mediterranean fever (p. 32)
Handigodu syndrome (p. 43)
Hereditary progressive arthro-ophthalmopathy (p. 46)
Hereditary vascular and articular calcification (p. 47)
Intermittent hydrarthrosis (p. 58)
Léri's pleonosteosis (p. 66)
Macrodystrophia lipomatosa (p. 70)
Mseleni joint disease (p. 77)
Osteochondromatosis (p. 92)
Pigmented villonodular synovitis (p. 97)
Progeria (p. 147)
Pseudoxanthoma elasticum (p. 105)
Relapsing polychondritis (p. 111)
Sarcoidosis (p. 119)
Sudeck's atrophy (p. 127)
Takayasu's disease (p. 134)
Temporomandibular arthropathy (p. 135)
Tietze's syndrome (p. 139)
Transient osteoporosis of the hip (p. 140)
Transient painful osteoporosis (p. 140)
Transient synovitis of the hip (p. 141)
Wegener's granulomatosis (p. 146)
Werner's syndrome (p. 147)
Xiphoid syndrome (p. 151)

Normality with Symptoms
Non-disease (p. 85)
Psychogenic rheumatism (p. 106)

Dietary
Fluorosis (p. 33)
Kashin-Beck disease (p. 64)
Scurvy (p. 122)

Soft-tissue Syndromes simulating Arthritis
Back-pocket sciatica (p. 11)
Camptodactyly (p. 16)
Carpal tunnel syndrome (p. 22)
Compression neuropathies (p. 22)
Deep-vein thrombosis (p. 24)
Dupuytren's contracture (p. 26)
Frozen shoulder (p. 34)
Hereditary angio-oedema (p. 45)
Jumper's knee (p. 61)
Knuckle-pad syndrome (p. 64)
Lymphoedema praecox (p. 70)
Morton's metatarsalgia (p. 76)
Myositis ossificans (p. 82)
Neuralgic amyotrophy (p. 82)
Osgood-Schlatter's disease (p. 88)
Painful fat knees (p. 94)
Sever's disease (p. 124)
Shoulder-hand syndrome (p. 125)
Tennis elbow (p. 137)
Traveller's ankle (p. 142)
Trochanteric syndrome (p. 142)

Pharmacological
For classification *see* p. 24
See also Drug-induced S. L. E. (p. 26)
See also Serum sickness (p. 124)

ARTHRITIS WITH DISEASE OF OTHER MAJOR SYSTEMS

Endocrine
Acromegaly (p. 1)
Hyperparathyroidism (p. 54)
Hypothyroidism (p. 56)
Idiopathic hypoparathyroidism (p. 56)
Thyroid acropachy (p. 138)

Haematological
Haemophilia (p. 42)
Leukaemia, acute (p. 67) and chronic (p. 68)
Sickle-cell disease (p. 126)

Neurological
Hemiplegia (p. 43)
Neuropathic (p. 83)

Gastro-enterological
Chronic active hepatitis (p. 45)
Cirrhosis of the liver (p. 19)
Crohn's disease (p. 28)
Enteropathic synovitis (p. 28)
Idiopathic steatorrhoea (p. 57)
Intestinal by-pass for obesity (p. 60)
Pancreatitis and pancreatic carcinoma (p. 95)
Ulcerative colitis (p. 28)
Whipple's disease (p. 148)

CLASSIFICATION OF THE ARTHROPATHIES

Dermatological

Acne arthralgia (p. 1)
Angiokeratoma corporis diffusum (p. 6)
Cutaneous polyarteritis nodosa (p. 23)
Erythema multiforme (p. 30)
Erythema nodosum (p. 31)
Nail-patella syndrome (p. 82)
Psoriatic arthropathy (p. 105)
Pyoderma gangrenosum (p. 107)
Sweet's syndrome (p. 128)
Urticaria (p. 144)

Neoplastic

For classification *see* p. 71
See also:—
Atrial myxoma (p. 10)
Carcinoid syndrome (p. 16)
Carcinoma arthritis (p. 16)
Haemangioma (p. 41)

Leukaemia, acute (p. 67) and chronic (p. 68)
Myeloma (p. 81)
Pseudohypertrophic osteo-arthropathy
(p. 104)
Synovioma (p. 129)

Renal Transplantation and Haemodialysis
(p. 112)

Arthritis Secondary to Disease of Bone
Avascular necrosis (p. 10)
Chondrodysplasic rheumatism (p. 18)
François syndrome (p. 33)
Melorheostosis (p. 72)
Osteochondritis dissecans (p. 91)
Osteomalacia and rickets (p. 92)
Paget's disease (p. 93)
Periostitis deformans (p. 96)
Perthes disease (p. 96)
Thiemann's disease (p. 137)

INTRODUCTION

To make a diagnosis, the human brain functions as a computer, fitting the presence and absence of clinical features to the known characteristics of diseases. In order to make the correct diagnosis, it is therefore necessary to know as much about the rarest disease as the commonest, and this book aims to provide such information. It is not intended for reading, but for consultation when information is required. It is not a textbook, and having no pictures, makes no attempt to replace the experience of seeing patients which is essential to learning rheumatology.

THE INFORMATION IS ORGANIZED AS FOLLOWS:

Definition of disease X, including aetiology if known, and inheritance.

Incidence or prevalence of arthritis in disease X; age and sex, type and stage of disease X in which arthritis is particularly seen; family history; persons specially predisposed.

Joints affected. How many? Which? How often? Symmetrical or asymmetrical? Migratory?

Symptoms, including speed of onset and precipitating factors.

Signs.

Course of the arthritis and of the underlying disease. If episodic, frequency, regularity, and duration of attacks. Effect of treatment.

Associations, radiological findings, and useful *laboratory tests.*

Treatment.

Where possible, the exact frequency of any occurrence is given; this is based on a survey of the literature and modified by personal experience. Where it is not possible to give exact frequencies, the following approximations are used:

Usual:	at least 90 per cent
Common:	at least 70 per cent
Often:	40–70 per cent
Occasional:	10–40 per cent
Uncommon:	less than 10 per cent
Rare:	less than 1 per cent

One or two recent references are given where possible, as a starting point for those seeking further information.

INCIDENCE OF ARTHROPATHIES

So that a correct diagnosis may be made, the frequency of different arthropathies must be known, as well as their clinical features and the clinical features of the case. For example, though rheumatoid arthritis is usually polyarticular, it is a much more likely cause of arthritis of a single joint than pigmented villonodular synovitis. The exact frequency of many diseases is not known, but in rheumatological practice in England one might expect to see the arthropathies in the following proportions:—

Several times each week:
  Rheumatoid arthritis.
  Osteoarthritis.
  Normality with symptoms (psychogenic rheumatism or non-disease).
  Frozen shoulder, tennis elbow, and other varieties of soft-tissue rheumatism.
  Traumatic and occupational arthropathies.

Several times each month:
  Gout. Pyrophosphate arthropathy.
  Psoriatic arthropathy.
  Reiter's disease.
  Ankylosing spondylitis.
  Polymyalgia rheumatica.
  Drug-induced arthropathies.

Several times each year:
  Systemic lupus erythematosus.
  Polyarteritis nodosa.
  Polymyositis and dermatomyositis.
  Septic arthritis.
  Tuberculous arthritis.
  Scleroderma.
  Juvenile chronic arthritis.
  Palindromic rheumatism.
  Pseudohypertrophic osteoarthropathy and other arthropathies associated with malignant
    disease.
  Neuropathic joints.
  Shoulder–hand syndrome.
  Ankylosing vertebral hyperostosis.
  Arthritis associated with ulcerative colitis, rubella, sarcoidosis, and erythema nodosum.

The remainder are rare and should be diagnosed with caution. In other parts of the world, and in other specialities such as paediatrics, the relative incidence of the arthropathies may be quite different.

CAUSES OF JOINT PAIN[1]

1. *Joint disease*: The arthropathies.

2. *Bone disease*: Fractures, primary or secondary tumours, osteochondritis, osteomyelitis, etc.

3. *Soft-tissue lesions*:
   Sprains and strains.
   Tenosynovitis.
   Overuse syndromes.
   'Soft-tissue rheumatism.'
   Direct trauma.
   Bursitis.

4. *Arthralgia*: Defined as joint pain in the absence of objective evidence of joint disease. This occurs in a variety of conditions, including:
   A. THE ARTHROPATHIES, either preceding the development of local signs or in some conditions in which there may be no local signs. Important examples are polymyalgia rheumatica and temporal arteritis, systemic lupus erythematosus and polyarteritis nodosa.
   B. INFECTIONS, particularly viral and rickettsial.
   Virus infections: influenza (25 per cent of cases), glandular fever, psittacosis, yellow fever, and sandfly fever.
   Rickettsial infections: all types of typhus.
   Bacterial infections: septicaemia, subacute bacterial endocarditis, typhoid and salmonella infections, and brucellosis.
   Spirochaetal infections: secondary syphilis, leptospirosis, and relapsing fever.
   Protozoal and metazoal infections: kala-azar and many other tropical, febrile conditions.
   C. DRUGS (*see* p. 24), immunization, and allergies.
   D. PROTEIN ABNORMALITIES, e.g., mixed IgG IgM cryoglobulinaemia.[2]

5. *Referred pain* is particularly common in the shoulder joint when it may be due to:
   A. Abdominal conditions: liver abscess, subphrenic abscess, gall-bladder disease, peritonitis.
   B. Oesophageal conditions: hiatus hernia.
   C. Cardiac conditions: myocardial ischaemia.
   D. Neurological conditions: cervical cord or brachial plexus lesions.
   E. Pulmonary conditions: apical tumours, pleurisy, pneumothorax.
   Pain in the knee is often due to hip disease.

6. *Psychogenic*: Aches and pains are common in normal people, particularly women. Some have a tendency to joint pains from childhood which continue throughout life, often related to weather conditions (so-called 'rheumatism'). Joint pain may be a manifestation of psychological disturbance and rheumatism may become a source of complaint in anxious or neurotic patients.

REFERENCES

[1] HART, F. D. (1970), *Annals of Physical Medicine*, **10**, 257.
[2] MELTZER, M., and others (1966), *American Journal of Medicine*, **40**, 837.

HISTORY

1. BACKGROUND INFORMATION. Age, sex, race, occupation.
2. MAIN COMPLAINT
   a. When did it start?
   b. How did it start? (Sudden, gradual, time of day.)
   c. Precipitating factors:
   Trauma, excessive or unusual activity.
   Infection—sore throat, urethral discharge, septic lesions such as boils.
   Unusual sexual exposure.
   Foreign travel.
   Contact with infectious diseases.
   Drugs, vaccination, injections, surgery.
   Excess of food or alcohol.
   Exposure to sunlight or cold.
   Emotional stress.
   d. Pattern of joint involvement:
   How many joints?
   First joint or joints affected.
   Subsequent joints affected.
   Pattern of development: episodic, migratory, additive, simultaneous.
   Symmetry or asymmetry.
   Severity—worst affected joint or joints.
   e. Time pattern. If symptoms are persistent:
   Relation to time of day.
   Night pain and interference with sleep.
   Morning stiffness.
   If symptoms are episodic:
   Frequency of episodes.
   Regularity of episodes.
   Duration of episodes.
   f. Aggravating and relieving factors:
   Effect of rest and exercise, activity and immobility, and treatments.
   g. Resultant problems:
   Extent of disability; note ability to carry out essential tasks of daily living, washing, bathing, eating, toilet activities, walking, sitting and standing, stairs etc.
   Ability to follow usual occupation.
   Particular disabilities, e.g., painful movements or difficult activities.
3. ASSOCIATED SYMPTOMS
   a. General. Malaise. Fatigue.
   b. Specific. Fever. Rash. Diarrhoea and other abdominal symptoms.
   Weight loss. Pains elsewhere. Symptoms referable to other systems.
4. PAST MEDICAL HISTORY
   Rheumatic fever.   Psoriasis.
   Tuberculosis.   History of arthritis in childhood.
   Record details of past complaints, investigations, etc.—frequent fruitless investigation and polysymptomatosis are characteristic accompaniments of psychogenic rheumatism.
5. FAMILY HISTORY
   Enquire particularly for ankylosing spondylitis, psoriasis, Behçet's disease, gout, rheumatoid arthritis, ulcerative colitis and Crohn's disease.
6. SOCIAL PSYCHOLOGICAL AND DOMESTIC DETAILS
   Work and home circumstances.
   Unusual or deficient diet.
   Possibly contributory emotional and social problems.
   Mental attitude. Motivation.
7. DRUGS AND OTHER TREATMENTS
   Present treatment for arthritis—dose and régime.
   Past treatment; benefit; side effects; outcome (if stopped, why?).
   Drugs for other diseases.

EXAMINATION

1. GENERAL
   Appearance: well or ill?
   Obvious diagnosis such as myxoedema or acromegaly.
   Pallor, pigmentation and skin rashes.
   Posture.
   Gait.
2. EXAMINATION OF JOINTS
   a. *Appearance:*
      Overlying skin: colour and consistency (smooth, shiny etc.).
      Swelling?
      Resting position. Deformities.
   b. *Palpation:*
      Warmth?
      Nature of swelling. Effusion, soft tissue or bony swelling.
      Tenderness. Localization and severity.
   c. *Active movement:*
      Range.
      Pain?
      Crepitus.
      Power.
   d. *Passive movement:*
      Range.
      Pain?
      Crepitus.
      Stability.
      Are deformities correctible?
3. SOFT TISSUES.
   Muscles.   Power. Wasting.
   Tendons.   Palpable abnormality (thickening, localized swelling): Tenderness. Crepitus.
                 Functional abnormalities such as triggering. Rupture.
   Bursae.   Swelling. Tenderness. Signs of inflammation.
   Ligaments.   Tenderness. Stability.
   Tendon sheath swelling?
   Nodules. Tophi, etc.
4. COMPLETE PHYSICAL EXAMINATION ESSENTIAL. Look particularly for:
   1. Non-articular features of rheumatoid arthritis, nodules, peripheral neuropathy, lymphadenopathy etc.
   2. Tophi.
   3. Rashes. Remember that psoriasis may be minimal and hidden in the natal cleft or scalp. Look at hands for vasculitic lesions. Many other arthropathies are associated with skin lesions including purpura, erythema nodosum, scleroderma, rubella and dermatomyositis.
   4. Finger clubbing or other evidence of malignant disease such as hepatomegaly or lymphnode enlargement.
   5. Temporal arteritis.
   6. Evidence of infection from boils to tuberculosis. Examine genital tract if suspicious of gonorrhoea or Reiter's disease.
   7. Splenomegaly and lymphadenopathy.
   8. Evidence of gastrointestinal disease including perianal disease such as fissure or fistula associated with ulcerative colitis.
   9. Fever.

JOINT PUNCTURE

INDICATIONS

1. Diagnostic, particularly suspicion of septic or infective arthritis and crystal deposition diseases (gout and pyrophosphate arthropathy).

2. For intra-articular injection of (a) steroids, particularly in chronic inflammatory arthritis for a single joint which is persistently painful despite rest and anti-inflammatory drugs or to aid mobilization of a joint, or (b) antibiotics, undesirable and unnecessary except for those antibiotics which are too toxic to give parenterally, e.g., polymyxin B.

3. To aspirate synovial fluid in septic arthritis; this is sometimes useful with very large effusions, haemarthroses, and pyrophosphate arthropathy.

4. For synovial biopsy, particularly for diagnosis of either rheumatoid arthritis or tuberculosis.

RISKS

1. Infection; about 1 in 10,000 if proper precautions are taken.

2. Destructive changes following repeated intra-articular steroid injection.

3. Inflammation due to injection of crystalline steroid preparations.

PRECAUTIONS

1. Strict asepsis.

2. Not more than three steroid injections in any joint.

3. Warn the patient (a) to report at once if the joint becomes more painful, and (b) to rest for at least 24 hours, and to avoid excessive weight-bearing for 3 weeks.

SITE: Descriptions such as 'above' and 'downwards' refer to the patient in position for injection and not to standard anatomical positions.

JOINT	PATIENT	NEEDLE ENTERS
Knee	Lying, knee slightly flexed	Medial side, below the patella, needle directed laterally and slightly downwards
Ankle	Lying	Just in front of, and medial to, medial malleolus, needle directed downwards and slightly laterally
Hip	Lying	2 cm. below the inguinal ligament just lateral to the femoral artery, needle directed downwards and slightly medially
Shoulder	Sitting; arm resting by side	Just below the coracoid process, needle directed posteriorly
Elbow	Sitting; elbow flexed to 90°	Behind and 1 cm. below the lateral epicondyle, needle directed medially, and slightly towards the hand
Wrist	Sitting; hand resting palm downwards	Just distal to ulnar styloid process, needle directed downwards
M.C.P. or P.I.P. joints	Sitting; hand resting palm downwards	Medial or lateral side of dorsal surface, needle directed downwards and laterally or medially

DOSE: Hydrocortisone or prednisolone, 25–50 mg. (1–2 ml.) for knee and other large joints, 12·5 mg. for small joints of hands and temporomandibular joint.

SYNOVIAL FLUID

After aspiration note volume, colour, clarity, turbidity, blood-staining, and viscosity. Divide as follows:

2 ml. in a tube containing EDTA for cell count and differential	At least 1 ml. in a sterile container for microscopy and culture. Ask for urgent Gram stain or special culture media if indicated	Remainder: examine a wet film for crystals under polarized light. Note presence or absence of clot formation after standing

RESULTS: The characteristics of synovial fluid depend upon the presence or absence of inflammation of synovium. *Non-inflammatory fluid* is clear, viscous, fails to clot on standing, and contains less than 1000 cells $\times 10^9$/dl., predominantly mononuclear. *Inflammatory fluid* is non-viscous, may clot, and contains an increased number of white blood-cells. These changes may be slight or gross, depending on the severity of the inflammatory process. Fluid with a high white-cell count is turbid and this does not necessarily mean that it is septic. The characteristics of inflammatory and non-inflammatory fluid are summarized in the following table. Synovial fluid characteristics in individual arthropathies are shown with other laboratory features of the conditions.

	NON-INFLAMMATORY	INFLAMMATORY		
	E.g., Normal Fluid or Traumatic Arthritis	Rheumatoid Arthritis	Septic Arthritis	Gout or Pyrophosphate Arthropathy
Appearance	Clear	Often turbid	Turbid	Clear with flakes of fibrin
Colour	Yellow	Yellow/green	Brown/green	Yellow
Viscosity	High	Low	Low	Low
Clots	No	Yes	Yes	Yes
Approx. W.B.C. ($\times 10^9$/dl.)	1,000	30,000	100,000	10,000
Predominant cell	Mononuclears	Neutrophils	Neutrophils	Neutrophils
Crystals	No	No	No	Yes
Culture	Sterile	Sterile	Positive	Sterile

IDENTIFICATION OF CRYSTALS. Uric acid crystals are needle-shaped and strongly negatively birefringent (blue across the plane of the first-order red compensator); pyrophosphate crystals have square ends and are weakly positively birefringent (blue along the plane of the compensator).

SPECIAL TESTS
1. Complement levels are low in rheumatoid arthritis and high in Reiter's disease.
2. Latex tests parallel serum titres in patients with rheumatoid arthritis; there is a high incidence of false positives in other conditions and the test has little diagnostic value.

DRUGS USED FOR RHEUMATIC DISEASES

CLASSIFICATION

Group 1: *Simple Analgesics* to be used in single doses by mouth in the dosage shown.
Effective: placebo—very safe—red the best colour.
A little more effective: paracetamol (1 g.), dihydrocodeine (60 mg.), mefenamic acid (500 mg.), pentazocine (50 mg.), dextropropoxyphene (65 mg.).
More effective still: aspirin (600 mg.); paracetamol with dextropropoxyphene (Distalgesic) 2 tablets; aspirin with codeine (Codis) 2 tablets.

Group 2: *Non-steroidal Analgesic Anti-inflammatory Drugs.*
Propionic acid derivatives and similar compounds.
Propionic acid derivatives:
fenoprofen (600 mg. q.d.s.), flurbiprofen (50 mg. q.d.s.), ketoprofen (50 mg. t.d.s.), ibuprofen (300 mg. q.d.s.), naproxen (250 mg. b.d.).
Compounds like propionic acid derivatives:
Sulindac (100 mg. b.d.), Azapropazone (300 mg. q.d.s.).
flufenamic acid (200 mg. t.d.s.), alclofenac (1 g. t.d.s.).
Aspirin and similar compounds:
Aspirin (3·6 g. daily or more).
Indomethacin (25 mg. t.d.s. and up to 100 mg. *nocte*).
Phenylbutazone (or oxyphenbutazone) (100 mg. t.d.s.).

Group 3: *Pure Anti-inflammatory Drugs:* corticosteroids and ACTH.
Prednisolone suitable for most purposes—dose varies with the condition treated—*see under* individual arthropathies.

Group 4: *Drugs with a specific Action in Particular Conditions:*
Rheumatoid arthritis: penicillamine, gold, levamisole, immunosuppressive drugs (azathioprine, chlorambucil, cyclophosphamide), and chloroquine.
Gout: colchicine, allopurinol, and uricosuric drugs.
Others: *see under* individual arthropathies.

NON-SPECIFIC TREATMENT FOR RELIEF OF RHEUMATIC SYMPTOMS

Milder conditions. The following scheme is particularly suitable for minor musculoskeletal syndromes including soft-tissue rheumatism, osteoarthritis, and milder cases of rheumatoid arthritis. In these conditions, a powerful anti-inflammatory effect is not required and the use of major anti-inflammatory drugs with toxic side-effects is not justified at least until the safer drugs have been tried.
1. For mild cases or intermittent pain, use single doses of simple analgesics (group 1) taken 'on demand'. Start with paracetamol and try distalgesic or aspirin if this is not sufficient.
2. If regular treatment is required, start with a propionic acid derivative. If one doesn't work, try another—some patients respond to only one and there is no way of predicting which one.
3. Supplement with single doses of simple analgesics.
4. For pain at night or morning stiffness, add indomethacin 75–100 mg. *nocte* by mouth or suppository.
5. If symptoms are not controlled, try full doses of aspirin, indomethacin, or phenylbutazone. Supplement with simple analgesics and indomethacin at night.

Severe conditions with prominent inflammation. In these conditions the major anti-inflammatory drugs are most suitable:
Severe active rheumatoid arthritis: full doses of aspirin with indomethacin at night.
Ankylosing spondylitis: indomethacin or phenylbutazone.
Gout: indomethacin, phenylbutazone, or colchicine.
See also under individual arthropathies.

FAILURE TO RESPOND

These drugs are effective within a week and there is no justification for continuing treatment which is ineffective. Therefore:
1. Review the diagnosis and consider other forms of therapy such as local steroid injection. Oral anti-inflammatory drugs are entirely unsuitable for some conditions such as tennis elbow.
2. Consider specific therapy if available. Patients with rheumatoid arthritis and (*a*) uncontrolled symptoms despite optimal anti-inflammatory therapy, (*b*) developing deformities, or (*c*) evidence of radiological progression should be treated with penicillamine or gold (see p. 116).
Steroids should not be regarded as non-specific therapy for the relief of rheumatic symptoms. They should be used only for particular conditions such as polymyalgia rheumatica (*see under* individual arthropathies).

ABBREVIATIONS

ACTH:	Adrenocorticotrophin	I.P.:	Interphalangeal
A.N.F.:	Antinuclear factor	kg.:	Kilograms
ASO:	Anti-streptolysin O	LDH:	Lactic dehydrogenase
b.d.:	To be given twice daily	L.E.:	Lupus erythematosus
cf.:	Compare	M.:	Male
cm.:	Centimetres	M.C.P.:	Metacarpophalangeal
c.mm.:	Cubic millimetre	M.T.P.:	Metatarsophalangeal
C.M.C.:	Carpometacarpal	PBI	Protein-bound iodine
C.N.S.:	Central nervous system	P.I.P.:	Proximal interphalangeal
C.S.F.:	Cerebrospinal fluid	p.r.n.:	To be given when required
CXR:	Chest X-ray	q.d.s.:	To be given four times daily
D.I.P.:	Distal interphalangeal	S.L.E.:	Systemic lupus erythematosus
DNA:	Deoxyribonucleic acid	t.d.s.:	To be given three times daily
E.C.G.:	Electrocardiograph	T.P.I.:	*Treponema pallidum* immobilization
E.M.G.:	Electromyograph		test
E.S.R.:	Erythrocyte sedimentation rate	W.B.C.:	White blood-count
F.:	Female	W.R.:	Wassermann reaction
F.H.:	Family history	XR:	X-ray appearances
g.:	Grammes	>:	Greater than
I.M.:	Intramuscular	<:	Less than

RHEUMATOLOGICAL JARGON

Monarticular:	Affecting one joint.
Polyarticular (polyarthritis):	Affecting more than one joint.
Oligoarticular:	Affecting only a few joints.
Episodic:	Two or more attacks of arthritis with periods of complete remission between them.
Acute:	Severe and rapidly reaching a peak.
Chronic:	Lasting for a very long time.
Bilateral:	Affecting the same joints on both sides of the body.
Symmetrical:	Affecting the same joints to the same extent on both sides of the body.
Migratory:	Arthritis moving from joint to joint, the first affected joint becoming normal when the second is involved.
Additive:	Arthritis moving from joint to joint, the first affected joint persisting with the involvement of the second and subsequent joints.
Simultaneous:	Arthritis affecting a number of joints, all of which are affected from the beginning of the illness.
Arthralgia:	Joint pain without visible or palpable abnormality.
Large joints:	Hips, knees, ankles, shoulders, elbows, and wrists.
Small joints:	M.C.P., M.T.P., and interphalangeal joints of hands and feet.

BACK PAIN

Back pain is a very common clinical problem. It may be brought about by pathological processes affecting:[1]

1. Nerve endings in capsules of apophyseal joint, spinal ligaments, vertebral periosteum, and attached fasciae and tendons, dura mater and epidural adipose tissue, walls of arterioles supplying vertebral cancellous bone, and walls of epidural and paravertebral veins.
2. Afferent fibres in dorsal nerve roots and their branches.
3. Spasm of paravertebral muscles.
4. Pain receptor systems in visceral tissues segmentally innervated from dorsal spinal nerve roots.

Causes[2] are numerous and are listed below. It has to be admitted that in many cases the cause is not found, but it is important to consider the possibility that back pain in a particular patient is due to some serious underlying disease such as myeloma and this is the purpose of the following classification. Back pain may also be normal, for example after unaccustomed gardening by an atrophic desk-bound tycoon. It is also a common symptom of psychological disturbance and may start or become a source of complaint as a result of some social, domestic or matrimonial trouble. When back pain is normal or psychogenic, not the result of disease, it is particularly important to make the correct diagnosis since an inappropriate diagnosis of disease (such as 'arthritis of the spine' often diagnosed on the basis of degenerative changes on X-ray which are common before and universal after the age of 55) may itself be disabling. Apart from normality, psychological disorders, and 'situational states', most cases of backache are due to traumatic, degenerative and mechanical conditions, in which it is often impossible to make an exact diagnosis.

1. *Normality. Non-disease* (p. 85).
2. *Psychogenic* (p. 106).
3. *Non-infective, traumatic, degenerative and mechanical disorders:*

Bad posture and strain	Disc lesions
Injuries	Osteoarthritis (p. 89)
Fatigue	Spondylolisthesis
Obesity	Sacro-iliac strain (p. 118)
Pregnancy	Neuropathic joint (p. 83)

4. *Generalized diseases of bone and metabolic disorders:*

Osteoporosis	Ochronosis (p. 83)
Osteomalacia (p. 92)	Gaucher's disease (p. 37)
Hyperparathyroidism (p. 54)	Fluorosis
Paget's disease (p. 93)	Hypophosphataemic spondylopathy (p. 55)
Acromegaly (p. 1)	Idiopathic hypoparathyroidism (p. 56)
Renal osteodystrophy	

5. *Infections localized to the spine:*
   Bacterial: Staphylococcal osteomyelitis and septic infections of the spine; Tuberculosis (p. 143); Brucellosis (p. 14); Typhoid (p. 144) and other *Salmonella* infections (p. 118); Leptospirosis (p. 146); Syphilis (p. 130) and Yaws (p. 152).
   Fungal: Histoplasmosis (p. 49); Blastomycosis (p. 13); Coccidioidomycosis (p. 21); African histoplasmosis (p. 3) and others (p. 35).
6. *Inflammatory conditions of the spine:*

Ankylosing spondylitis (p. 7)	Reiter's disease (p. 110)
Pyrophosphate arthropathy (p. 108)	Relapsing polychondritis (p. 111)
Sarcoidosis (p. 119)	Rheumatoid arthritis affecting the neck
Yersinia arthritis (p. 152)	(p. 114)
Polymyalgia rheumatica (p. 101)	

7. *Tumours*: primary or secondary, benign or malignant, affecting the cord or surrounding structures. See also myeloma (p. 81).
8. *Intrathoracic and cardiovascular*: aortic aneurysm, carcinoma of bronchus or oesophagus.
9. *Gastro-intestinal*: pancreatitis, carcinoma of pancreas or stomach, gall-stones, peptic ulcer.
10. *Renal*: pyelonephritis, stone or carcinoma of kidney, papillary necrosis.
11. *Gynaecological*: dysmenorrhoea, childbirth, pelvic infection or carcinoma, endometriosis.
12. *Generalized infections*: (the 'febrile' back) occurring in a variety of fevers from influenza to dengue and acute febrile lumbago in infective endocarditis (*see* p. 57).
13. *Blood disorders*: Sickle-cell crises (*see* p. 126) and acute haemolytic states.

REFERENCES

[1] WYKE, B. D. (1970), *Rheumatology and Physical Medicine*, **10**, 356.

[2] HART, F. D. (1973), *French's Index of Differential Diagnosis*, 10th ed. Bristol: John Wright.

RANGE OF MOVEMENT OF JOINTS

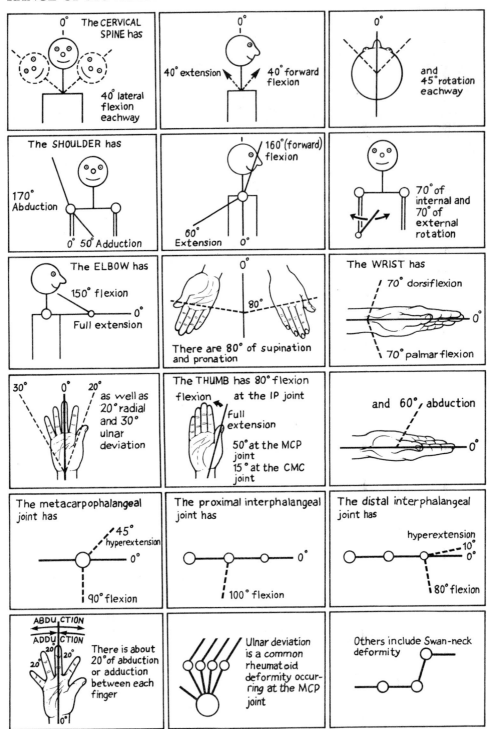

The CERVICAL SPINE has 0°

40° extension   40° forward flexion

40° lateral flexion eachway

0°   and 45° rotation eachway

The SHOULDER has

170° Abduction

0° 50° Adduction

160° (forward) flexion

60° Extension   0°

70° of internal and 70° of external rotation

The ELBOW has

150° flexion

0° Full extension

0°   80°

There are 80° of supination and pronation

The WRIST has

70° dorsiflexion   0°

70° palmar flexion

30°   0°   20°

as well as 20° radial and 30° ulnar deviation

The THUMB has 80° flexion at the IP joint

flexion   Full extension

50° at the MCP joint

15° at the CMC joint

and 60°, abduction

0°

The metacarpophalangeal joint has

45° hyperextension   0°

90° flexion

The proximal interphalangeal joint has

0°

100° flexion

The distal interphalangeal joint has

hyperextension 10°   0°

80° flexion

ABDUCTION

ADDUCTION

20°   20°

20°   20°

0°

There is about 20° of abduction or adduction between each finger

Ulnar deviation is a common rheumatoid deformity occurring at the MCP joint

Others include Swan-neck deformity

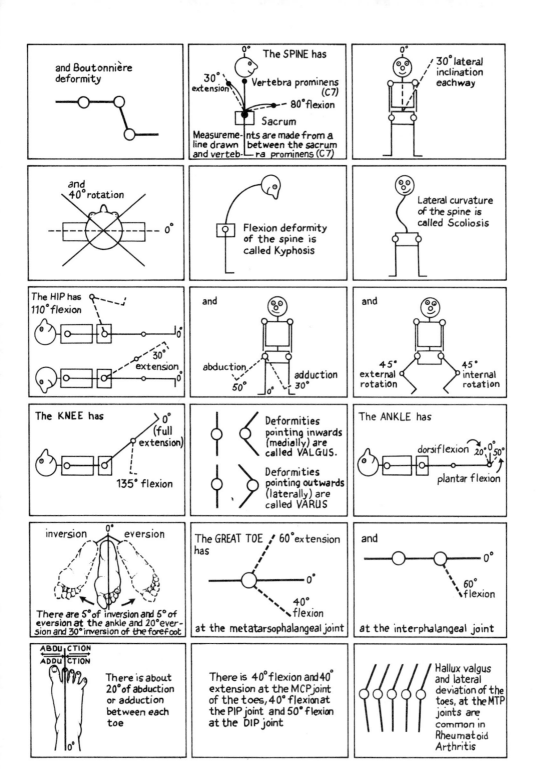

and Boutonnière deformity

The SPINE has
30° extension
Vertebra prominens (C7)
80° flexion
Sacrum
Measureme-nts are made from a line drawn between the sacrum and verteb-ra prominens (C7)

30° lateral inclination eachway

and 40° rotation
0°

Flexion deformity of the spine is called Kyphosis

Lateral curvature of the spine is called Scoliosis

The HIP has 110° flexion
30° extension

and
abduction 50°
adduction 30°

and
45° external rotation
45° internal rotation

The KNEE has
0° (full extension)
135° flexion

Deformities pointing inwards (medially) are called VALGUS.

Deformities pointing outwards (laterally) are called VARUS

The ANKLE has
dorsiflexion 20° 0° 50°
plantar flexion

inversion 0° eversion
There are 5° of inversion and 5° of eversion at the ankle and 20° ever-sion and 30° inversion of the forefoot

The GREAT TOE has
60° extension
0°
40° flexion
at the metatarsophalangeal joint

and
0°
60° flexion
at the interphalangeal joint

ABDUCTION
ADDUCTION
0°

There is about 20° of abduction or adduction between each toe

There is 40° flexion and 40° extension at the MCP joint of the toes, 40° flexion at the PIP joint and 50° flexion at the DIP joint

Hallux valgus and lateral deviation of the toes, at the MTP joints are common in Rheumatoid Arthritis

ACANTHOCHEILONEMA PERSTANS

A filarial worm infestation found in tropical Africa, South America, and New Guinea, which is usually asymptomatic, but may cause joint pain and swelling affecting one or many joints. There is eosinophilia and microfilariae are found in the blood.

REFERENCE

British Medical Journal (1969), **1**, 204.

ACNE ARTHRALGIA

Arthralgia may be associated with acne conglobata, a severe destructive variety of acne in which individual lesions join up to produce areas of necrosis, or ulceration with scab formation or haemorrhage, usually on the face or upper trunk.

It particularly affects adolescent boys who may present with arthralgia, particularly in the hips and other central joints. There may be limitation of movement but joints are otherwise normal. Attacks of arthralgia last for weeks or months, subside without residua, and only rarely recur. There is fever and the white cell count and E.S.R. may be raised. Treatment: (1) Aspirin and other symptomatic remedies. Steroids in severe cases which fail to respond to simpler measures. (2) Treatment of the acne with tetracycline and local ointments. The condition may be mediated by immune complexes since complement levels are reduced.

REFERENCE

LANE, J. M., and others (1976), *Journal of Bone and Joint Surgery*, **58A**, 673.

ACROMEGALY

A pituitary adenoma causing chronic over-production of growth hormone which in adults results in gradual enlargement of the bones of the head, hands, and feet.

Incidence
F. 3 : 2.
Commonest onset age 20–40.
50 per cent have arthropathy.

Joints affected
Finger joints, spine, and knees often.
Hips, shoulders, ankles, wrists, elbows occasionally.
Polyarticular; symmetrical.

Symptoms
Pain in back and affected joints.
Intermittent swelling.
Stiffness unusual.

Signs
1. Enlargement of joints due to synovial thickening and bony outgrowth.
2. Crepitus.
3. Recurrent effusion common.
4. Increased mobility in early stages; later restriction of movement in severely affected peripheral joints, but not spine.

Course
Intermittent episodes of pain lasting weeks or months.
May progress slowly or rapidly to severe disabling arthropathy, resembling late stages of osteoarthritis.

Associated features
1. Bilateral carpal tunnel syndrome in 40 per cent.
   Improves after hypophysectomy.
2. Other features of acromegaly, typical facies, large hands, hypertension, etc.
   Look for visual field changes.

XR
1. 'Tufting' of distal phalanges.
2. Increased joint space.
3. Bony outgrowth around joints ('lipping') especially bases of distal phalanges ('hooks') and spine.
4. Small areas of calcification of joint capsule and cartilage.
5. Thickened widely spaced bony trabeculae.
6. Enlarged pituitary fossa.
   No erosions.

1

ACROMEGALY (*continued*)

Laboratory
Confirm the diagnosis by insulin- and glucose-tolerance tests, growth hormone level.

Treatment
1. Analgesics.

2. Consider hypophysectomy but this has no effect on arthropathy.
3. Consider carpal tunnel decompression.
4. Surgery in advanced cases.
5. Bromocriptine may improve soft-tissue changes but not arthritis.

REFERENCES

BLUESTONE, R., and others (1971), *Annals of the Rheumatic Diseases*, 30, 243.

KELLGREN, J. H., and others (1952), *Quarterly Journal of Medicine*, 21, 405.

ACRO-OSTEOLYSIS

A group of conditions characterized by destruction and disappearance of bone. This may be primary or secondary to various joint diseases. Osteolysis of articulating surfaces occurs as a complication of rheumatoid arthritis, psoriatic arthropathy, avascular necrosis, and chronic infection. Osteolysis of distal phalanges of hands or feet occurs in scleroderma, Raynaud's disease, leprosy, and peripheral arterial obstruction. Acro-osteolysis may also be caused by polyvinyl chloride (P.V.C.). Patients develop Raynaud's phenomenon lytic bone lesions in the extremities and sometimes scleroderma-like changes in the skin (*see* p. 121). Primary osteolysis is of four types, all rare.

1. *Hereditary osteolysis*:[1] inherited as an autosomal dominant character.

Incidence
M. = F.
Onset about age 3.

Joints affected
Wrists and ankles.
Usually bilateral.

Symptoms
Joint pain and swelling.

Signs—course
In early stages, joints are warm, tender, and swollen with limitation of movement.
Later signs of inflammation disappear but stiffness and deformities appear over the years.
The condition stabilizes spontaneously in early adult life.

XR
Porosis of carpal and tarsal bones appears at about age 6, followed by localized destruction progressing to complete disappearance by age 30. There is concave deformity of the adjacent ends of long bones.

Laboratory
Normal E.S.R.
Latex test negative.

Treatment
Steroids give symptomatic relief but have no effect on the course of the disease. Splints may be useful to prevent deformity. Surgery to correct deformity when active stage is over.

2. *Osteolysis with nephropathy*:[2] a non-hereditary condition otherwise resembling hereditary osteolysis, beginning in childhood and usually affecting wrists and ankles, sometimes also hands, feet, and elbows. It is associated with progressive and ultimately fatal chronic glomerulo-nephritis.

3. *Gorham's disease* (Disappearing or Phantom Bone Disease):[3] a non-hereditary condition of both sexes, appearing at age 5–65 (peak 10–30). Any bone may be affected, usually at multiple sites, asymmetrical in distribution and often occurring after mild trauma. There is weakness and limitation of movement, but pain is mild or absent. The condition eventually stabilizes sometimes with a 'boneless' limb. Histology shows proliferation of thin-walled vessels.

ACRO-OSTEOLYSIS (*continued*)

4. *Distal osteolysis*:[4] inherited as an autosomal dominant character, appears between the ages of 8 and 32, and is characterized by progressive osteolysis of phalanges, metatarsals, or metacarpals with recurrent ulceration of the hands and feet, and sequestration of bone fragments. Fingers and toes may be lost, but the condition eventually heals.

REFERENCES

[1] SHURTLEFF, D. B. (1964), *Journal of the American Medical Association*, **188**, 363.

[2] TORG, J. S., and STEEL, H. S. (1968), *Journal of Bone and Joint Surgery*, **50A**, 1629.

[3] ABELL, J. M., and BADGLEY, C. E. (1961), *Journal of the American Medical Association*, **177**, 771.

[4] SCHINZ, H. R., and others (1951), *Roentgen—Diagnostics*, Vol. 1, p. 734. New York: Grune & Stratton.

ADENOVIRUS ARTHRITIS

An acute polyarthritis is rarely associated with adenovirus infection, the more common manifestations of which include upper respiratory tract infection, fever, malaise and myalgia. Severe pain with effusions in the knees lasting for a few days has been reported. Synovial fluid was inflammatory with a predominance of polymorphs. The diagnosis can only be confirmed in retrospect by the demonstration of rising antibody titres. Treatment: Aspirin or other anti-inflammatory drugs.

REFERENCE

PANUSH, R. S. (1974), *Arthritis and Rheumatism*, **17**, 534.

AFRICAN HISTOPLASMOSIS

Infection with the fungus *Histoplasma duboisii*, found in West Africa. The source and mechanism of infection are unknown. Disease may be localized to the skin or disseminated, giving rise to granulomatous or suppurative lesions in bones, joints, liver, spleen, or lymph-nodes. In contrast to histoplasmosis (*see* p. 49) lung involvement is rare.

Incidence
M. 2 : 1.
Any age, peak 10–20.
About 20 per cent have arthritis.

Joints affected
Any joint or spine.
Usually monarticular.

Clinical features
Painful swollen joint.

Course
Chronic, may lead to joint destruction.

Associations
1. Skin lesions: painless papules which become nodules and may ulcerate.
2. Rarely hepatosplenomegaly, lymphadenopathy, or bone lesions.
3. Spinal involvement occasionally causes paraplegia.

XR
Well-defined osteolytic areas in bone adjacent to the joint.

Laboratory
Diagnosis is made by microscopical examination and culture of exudate from skin lesions or biopsy material from joint.

Treatment
Amphotericin B.

REFERENCE

COCKSHOTT, W. P., and LUCAS, A. O. (1964), *Quarterly Journal of Medicine*, **33**, 223.

AGAMMAGLOBULINAEMIA

A rare disorder characterized by absence of gamma-globulin on electrophoresis and diminished ability to produce circulating antibodies in response to antigenic stimulation. There are two types: *congenital*, transmitted as a sex-linked, recessive character and occurring in male children, and *primary acquired*, non-hereditary and occurring in both sexes at any age. The arthropathy bears a superficial resemblence to rheumatoid arthritis but differs in the absence of erosions and rheumatoid factor. Patients with agammaglobulinaemia are also liable to develop septic arthritis.

Incidence

Age 2–10 (congenital type) or 10–50 (acquired type).
30 per cent have arthritis, less common with the acquired type.
Arthritis appears several years after onset of infections.

Joints affected

Polyarticular.
Commonly knees, P.I.P. and M.C.P. joints.
Often wrists, ankles, and elbows.
Occasionally shoulders and hips.
Often asymmetrical.

Symptoms

Pain, often mild, sometimes absent.
Swelling and stiffness.

Signs

Soft-tissue swelling, limitation of movement, tenderness, effusion, and synovial thickening.
Warmth or erythema rare.

Course

Mild; may be episodic or chronic with relapses and remissions.
Bacterial infections may be fatal.

Associations

1. Recurrent bacterial infections, e.g., meningitis, septicaemia, urinary infection.
2. Nodules, histologically resembling rheumatoid nodules found in 30 per cent of cases; occasionally bursitis or tenosynovitis.
3. Collagen disease, e.g., dermatomyositis or scleroderma.
4. Lymphoma.

XR

Usually normal.
Occasionally periarticular porosis.

Laboratory

Raised E.S.R.
Latex test negative.
Very low levels of immunoglobulins.
Synovial fluid: non-inflammatory.
Synovial biopsy: indistinguishable from rheumatoid arthritis.

Treatment

1. Anti-inflammatory drugs but not steroids.
2. Gamma-globulin.
3. Antibiotics for infections.

REFERENCES

Good, R. A., and others (1957), *Journal of Laboratory and Clinical Medicine*, 49, 343.

Janeway, C. A., and others (1956), *Transactions of the Association of American Physicians*, 69, 93.

AMOEBIASIS

Infection with *Entamoeba histolytica* manifests as dysentery and is sometimes complicated by hepatitis, rarely with abscesses in the liver and elsewhere. Arthritis is rare and is probably not due to direct infection of joints. It is polyarticular, symmetrical or asymmetrical, and sometimes migratory. The joints are painful and may be swollen. This is often but not always associated with diarrhoea, rectal bleeding, or hepatitis. Amoebae are found in fresh stools and the arthritis responds to metronidazole or emetine.

REFERENCE

Rappaport, E. M. (1951), *Annals of Internal Medicine*, 34, 1224.

AMYLOIDOSIS

Amyloid infiltration of joint capsule, synovium, and tendons which gives rise to a polyarthritis resembling rheumatoid arthritis. This is usually associated with multiple myeloma but may also occur in primary amyloidosis with no apparent cause. Distinction is difficult since plasma cells are increased in the marrow in both conditions. There may be associated amyloid infiltration in other 'primary' sites.

Incidence

M. = F.
Age 30–70, peak 50–60.
Rare complication of myeloma. May precede other manifestations by up to 3 years.

Joints affected

Polyarticular.
Commonly affects small joints of hands, wrists, shoulders, and knees.
Often elbows, ankles, hips, and feet.
Bilateral and symmetrical.

Symptoms

Pain, swelling, stiffness, and limitation of motion.
Morning stiffness.
Often profound weakness.

Signs

Joints are swollen (effusion and synovial thickening) and tender but not red or warm.

Course

Arthritis may progress to flexion deformities resembling rheumatoid arthritis.
The condition is usually fatal within 5 years.

Associations

1. Bilateral carpal tunnel syndrome occurs in 50 per cent.
2. Nodules occur in 70 per cent, resembling those of rheumatoid arthritis but showing amyloid on biopsy.
3. Infiltration of amyloid elsewhere may cause heart failure or peripheral neuropathy.
4. Other features of myeloma, bone pain, anaemia, etc.

XR

Periarticular osteoporosis.
Osteolytic lesions of myeloma particularly in skull and vertebrae found in 50 per cent.

Laboratory

Anaemia and raised E.S.R.
Hypercalcaemia (30 per cent).
Latex test usually negative.
Proteins; paraprotein with reduction in immunoglobulin levels in 50 per cent.
Bence-Jones proteinuria (85 per cent).
Synovial fluid: non-inflammatory.
Diagnosis confirmed by biopsy of synovium, carpal ligament, or nodules which show amyloid. Bone-marrow shows excess of plasma cells.

Treatment

Poor response to analgesic anti-inflammatory drugs. Carpal tunnel decompression if necessary. Steroids and melphelan may produce remission in cases with myeloma.

REFERENCES

GOLDBERG, A., and others (1964), *American Journal of Medicine*, 37, 653.

WIERNICK, P. H. (1972), *Medicine*, 51, 465.

ANAEROBIC INFECTION

Infection with anaerobic organisms (*Bacterioides*, *Sphaerophorus* or anaerobic streptococci) should be suspected in a case which resembles septic arthritis, but in which cultures of synovial fluid are sterile. Anaerobic culture should then be requested. Joint involvement is usually monarticular but the pattern is a little different from septic arthritis due to other organisms (*see* p. 123). The knee or hip is affected in 60 per cent, shoulder, sternoclavicular joint, or elbow in 45 per cent; others are rare. Treatment as for septic arthritis. The antibiotic of choice is either penicillin or tetracycline, depending on the organism.

REFERENCE

ZIMENT, I., and others (1969), *Arthritis and Rheumatism*, **12**, 627.

ANGIOKERATOMA CORPORIS DIFFUSUM (Fabry's Disease)

A rare hereditary disease, transmitted as a sex-linked, recessive character. Vacuolated cells containing glycolipid are seen in the walls of blood-vessels.

Incidence

Usually males; females rarely and mildly affected.
Onset in childhood.

Articular manifestations

1. Distal interphalangeal joints of the fingers are commonly affected by a degenerative arthropathy, bilateral and symmetrical. There is bony swelling and flexion deformity. The condition is mild.
2. Pain in the fingers or toes may be mistaken for arthritis, though it is not confined to the joints. It is often burning in character and exacerbated by heat or exertion. It may be episodic or constant with exacerbations associated with febrile episodes.
3. Avascular necrosis occurs rarely (*see* p. 10).

Course

Death is usual at age 30–50 from uraemia or heart failure.
Arthritis is a minor problem.

Associations

1. Skin lesions: clusters of dark-red lesions up to 4 mm. in diameter in a symmetrical distribution around the pelvis.
2. Premature cerebral vascular disease, hypertension, and myocardial infarction.
3. Proteinuria leading to uraemia.
4. Ankle oedema.
5. Corneal opacity.
6. Diarrhoea and bleeding piles.

XR

Degenerative changes in distal interphalangeal joints.

Laboratory

Raised E.S.R. in febrile episodes.
Skin biopsy confirms the diagnosis.
No biochemical abnormality.

Treatment

Symptomatic.

REFERENCE

WISE, D., and others (1962), *Quarterly Journal of Medicine*, **31**, 177.

ANKYLOSING SPONDYLITIS

A chronic condition of the spine and sacro-iliac joints in which early inflammatory changes are followed by progressive restriction of spinal movement associated with radiological calcification of spinal ligaments.

Incidence

Affects 0·4 per cent of males. M. 5 : 1.
Age at onset 15–30 but rarely earlier or later.
F.H. in 6 per cent.

Joints affected

Initially sacro-iliacs affected symmetrically and bilaterally with involvement of entire spine thereafter.
Shoulders and hips affected in 40 per cent; peripheral joints in 25 per cent, knees, commonest (15 per cent), also ankles (10 per cent), feet (5 per cent), wrists (5 per cent), and rarely fingers.
Ribs fuse on to vertebrae and transverse processes; sternomanubrial and sternoclavicular joints often affected.

Symptoms

Gradual onset of low backache and/or pain in both buttocks (pseudo-bilateral sciatica).
Morning stiffness.
15 per cent present with peripheral arthritis.

Signs

1. Restriction of all movements of spine.
2. Chest expansion reduced (< 5 cm.).
3. Bony points often tender (heels, sternum, ribs, pelvic brim, and ischial tuberosities).
4. Peripheral joints may be swollen and tender.

Course

Tendency for stiffness to increase in the first few years.
Subsequently chronic but tending to improve, though hip involvement may be disabling.

Associations

1. Iritis in 25 per cent.
2. Aortic incompetence (1 per cent).
   Cardiac conduction defects (8 per cent).
Rarely:
3. Amyloidosis.
4. Atlanto-axial subluxation or fractures of rigid segments of the spine which may be fatal.
5. Apical pulmonary fibrosis[5] resembling pulmonary tuberculosis, associated with recurrent episodes of pneumonitis and pleurisy.
6. Cauda equina syndrome:[6] sphincter disturbances, sensory loss in the perineum, and absent ankle-jerks.

XR

Changes best seen in sacro-iliac joints and spine (D.10 to L.2).
1. *Pelvis.* Sacro-iliac joints usually abnormal; sclerosis; blurring of joint outline; later obliteration. Ischial tuberosities roughened and show 'whiskering' with periosteal elevations. Symphysis pubis may be blurred.
2. *Spine.* Syndesmophytes; longitudinal ligamentous calcification eventually producing 'bamboo' spine; lytic lesions appear particularly at the upper anterior corners of vertebral bodies; squaring of vertebrae.

Laboratory

E.S.R. raised in 80 per cent; often mild anaemia.
Latex test negative.
Synovial fluid: inflammatory; W.B.C. up to $20,000 \times 10^9$/dl., mainly neutrophils.
Tissue antigen HLA B 27 found in 96 per cent.[7]

Treatment

1. Exercise and exercises to maintain as full mobility as possible.
2. Phenylbutazone and indomethacin helpful in this programme. Night cover important. Indomethacin 100 mg. on retiring (by mouth or suppository). Not steroids.
3. Surgery only rarely needed, usually hip replacement. Spinal (wedge lumbar) osteotomy for marked kyphosis.
4. Radiotherapy in conservative dosage helpful but carries small risk of leukaemia and best avoided.

Variants

1. A similar picture may occasionally be seen in Reiter's disease, psoriasis, ulcerative colitis, Crohn's disease, and rarely Whipple's disease, Behçet's syndrome and familial Mediterranean fever.
2. Juvenile chronic arthritis in boys may later lead to ankylosing spondylitis (*see* p. 63)
3. In women,[3] the disease tends to be mild with limited spinal involvement. Pregnancy has no effect.

ANKYLOSING SPONDYLITIS (*continued*)

REFERENCES

[1] CALABRO, J. J., and MALTZ, B. A. (1970), *New England Journal of Medicine*, **282**, 606.

[2] HART, F. D. (1955), *Annals of the Rheumatic Diseases*, **14**, 77.

[3] HART, F. D., and ROBINSON, K. (1959), *Annals of the Rheumatic Diseases*, **18**, 15.

[4] WILKINSON, M., and BYWATERS, E. G. L. (1958), *Annals of the Rheumatic Diseases*, **17**, 209.

[5] DAVIES, D. (1972), *Quarterly Journal of Medicine*, **41**, 395.

[6] MATTHEWS, W. B. (1968), *Journal of the Neurological Sciences*, **6**, 561.

[7] BREWERTON, D. A., and others (1973), *Lancet*, **1**, 904.

ANKYLOSING VERTEBRAL HYPEROSTOSIS (Zuckergusswirbelsaüle)

A condition of the elderly in which there is exuberant bony outgrowth from the spine. The condition must be distinguished from ankylosing spondylitis (*see* p. 7) which occurs in young adults, and causes pain, restriction of spinal movement, often peripheral joint involvement, sacro-iliitis, and distinct X-ray changes. The X-ray appearance must be distinguished from paraspinal ossification in psoriatic arthropathy (*see* p. 105).

Incidence
Usually males.
Age 50+.

Joints affected
Spine (dorsal particularly).
No peripheral joint involvement.

Symptoms
Often none, sometimes stiffness.
No pain.

Signs
Normal or slight restriction of spinal movement.
No kyphosis.

Course
Benign: non-progressive.

Associations
Diabetes mellitus (often).

XR
Lateral views of spine show large bony outgrowths arising from the anterolateral aspect of the vertebral body.
They may extend upwards producing a 'candle-flame' appearance or downwards producing a 'dripping candle-wax' appearance.
They often join to form a continuous sheet of bone anterior to the vertebral bodies.
Sacro-iliac joints normal.

Laboratory
Normal E.S.R., calcium, phosphates, and alkaline phosphatase.
Test urine for sugar.

Treatment
Not required.
Maintain mobility.

REFERENCE
FORESTIER, J., and ROTES-QUEROL, J. (1950), *Annals of the Rheumatic Diseases*, **9**, 321.

ARTHROGRYPOSIS MULTIPLEX CONGENITA

Rare non-hereditary congenital disorder characterized by stiff, deformed joints and muscle wasting. The deformities may resemble those of advanced arthritis.

Incidence
M. = F.
Present at birth.

Joints affected
Deformities usually bilateral.
All four limbs affected in 50 per cent; both lower limbs in 30 per cent; rarely both upper limbs; occasionally asymmetrical.

Clinical features
1. Painless deformities.
   Feet: equinovarus deformity (75 per cent).
   Knees: flexion deformity (60 per cent); extension deformity (20 per cent).
   Hips: flexion deformity (40 per cent); dislocation (40 per cent), often bilateral; flexion, abduction, and external rotation deformity (20 per cent).
   Elbow: flexion deformity (20 per cent); extension deformity (30 per cent).
   Wrists: flexion deformity (40 per cent); extension, pronation or supination (20 per cent).
   Fingers: flexion deformity (50 per cent); extension deformity (5 per cent).
   Thumb: adduction-flexion deformity (25 per cent).
   Others rare.
2. Joint stiffness.

Course
Non-progressive.
Severe disability usual but normal life span.

Associations
1. Muscle wasting. Reflexes may be absent.
2. Smooth uncreased skin.
3. Webs (50 per cent) may aggravate deformities.
4. 'Port-wine' stains in 15 per cent.
5. Mental deficiency is rare.

XR
No bone changes.

Laboratory
No characteristic biochemical or histological features.

Treatment
1. Correction of deformities as far as possible by plastering, braces, etc.
2. Surgery: release operations, wedge resection, osteotomy, or arthrodesis.

REFERENCES

GIBSON, D. A., and URS, N. D. K. (1970), *Journal of Bone and Joint Surgery*, **52B**, 483.
LLOYD-ROBERTS, G. C., and LETTIN, A. W. F. (1970), *Journal of Bone and Joint Surgery*, **52B**, 494.

MEAD, N. G., and others (1958), *Journal of Bone and Joint Surgery*, **40A**, 1285.

ATRIAL MYXOMA

Rare benign tumour which arises from the atrial wall and grows out to obstruct the orifice of the mitral or tricuspid valve. 75 per cent arise from the left atrium. The condition usually presents as a cardiac problem with shortness of breath, weakness or syncope, and signs of mitral or tricuspid stenosis which change from day to day. Rarely, it presents as a rheumatic illness with joint pains, Raynaud's phenomenon, and raised E.S.R. The occurrence of emboli may suggest subacute bacterial endocarditis.

Incidence
Adults; any age. F. 2 : 1.
Arthritis is rare.

Joints affected
Polyarticular.
Small joints of hands, knees, or ankles particularly.
Bilateral and symmetrical.

Symptoms
Pain and swelling.
Malaise; loss of weight.

Signs
Often none.
Sometimes soft-tissue swelling or effusion.

Courses
Chronic.
Complete remission follows removal of tumour.
No residua.

Associations
1. Signs and symptoms of atrial myxoma (*see above*) particularly murmurs of mitral or tricuspid stenosis which are heard only intermittently.
2. Pulmonary or systemic emboli.
3. Raynaud's phenomenon.

XR
Normal.

Laboratory
Raised E.S.R.

Treatment
Removal of myxoma.

REFERENCE

CURREY, H. L. F., and others (1967), *British Medical Journal*, 1, 547.

AVASCULAR NECROSIS

A group of conditions in which bone infarction is not associated with sepsis but is usually due to interference with blood-supply, either by abnormalities of the vessel wall such as arteritis, pressure on vessels from outside, trauma, thrombosis, or embolism. Clinical disease results only when the surface of a joint is involved, causing arthritis.

The condition may be:

1. *Traumatic*: e.g., following fractures of the neck of the femur.

2. *Secondary to existing arthropathies*: (*a*) Rheumatoid arthritis. (*b*) Psoriatic arthropathy. (*c*) Severe osteoarthritis. (*d*) Neuropathic joint.

3. *Secondary to systemic conditions*: (*a*) Caisson disease (decompression syndrome). (*b*) Sickle-cell disease, particularly sickle-cell thalassaemia and sickle-cell–haemoglobin C disease (*see* p. 126). (*c*) High-dose steroid therapy, e.g., after renal transplantation (*see* p. 112), and in Cushing's disease. (*d*) Systemic lupus erythematosus (*see* p. 132). (*e*) Alcoholism. (*f*) Gaucher's disease (*see* p. 37). (*g*) Pancreatitis. (*h*) Pregnancy. (*i*) Extensive burns. (*j*) Distant trauma, e.g., multiple injuries. (*k*) Endocarditis. (*l*) Giant-cell arteritis (*see* p. 101). (*m*) Angiokeratoma corporis diffusum (*see* p. 6). (*n*) Radiation. (*o*) Scleroderma (*see* p. 121). (*p*) Diabetes mellitus. (*q*) Polycythaemia rubra vera. (*r*) Electrical injury. (*s*) Local steroids.

AVASCULAR NECROSIS (*continued*)

4. *Idiopathic Avascular Necrosis:* Most commonly occurs in the hips of middle-aged men (age (30–60, M.4 :1)—30 per cent have bilateral involvement. The second side may begin several years after the first. It may affect the knee when it occurs in elderly women and is almost always unilateral. Rarely the shoulder, elbow, wrist or ankle are involved. *See also* Perthes' disease (p. 96) and Thiemann's disease (p. 137).

Incidence
Any age, either sex, depending on underlying condition.

Joints affected
Usually one or both hips.
Rarely knees or shoulders.
30 per cent bilateral.

Symptoms
Pain of variable severity, often mild at onset.
Sudden or gradual onset.
Stiffness of affected joints.

Signs
Painful limitation of movement.
Recurrent large effusions if knees involved.

Course
Mild cases recover completely without residua within a few weeks or months.
Severe cases progress to complete destruction of joint requiring surgery.

Associations
Other features of underlying diseases.

XR
1. Small areas of infarction which may appear sclerotic or porotic.
2. Areas of joint surface collapse into underlying infarction producing flattening and irregularity.
3. Necrotic osteochondral fragments may separate partially or completely resembling osteochondritis dissecans (*see* p. 91); loose bodies may be seen.

Laboratory
Unhelpful except for diagnosis of underlying disease.

Treatment
1. In early cases, complete immobilization with no weight bearing.
2. Analgesics.
3. Surgery may be required, usually hip arthroplasty.

REFERENCES

DAVIDSON, J. K. (1976), *Aseptic Necrosis of Bone.* Amsterdam: Elsevier.
JONES, J. P., and ENGLEMAN, E. P. (1966), *Arthritis and Rheumatism,* 9, 728.
STOREY, G. O. (1968), *Proceedings of the Royal Society of Medicine,* 61, 961.

BACILLARY DYSENTERY (Shigella Infection)

May precede the development of Reiter's disease, particularly in certain parts of the world (*see* p. 110). Arthritis may occur without other manifestations of Reiter's disease, usually in the second or third week of the illness. One or more joints are affected, usually knees, elbows, wrists, or fingers; they are painful and swollen. Fever is common and there is sometimes tenosynovitis. The condition is unaffected by antibiotics and lasts for weeks or months, eventually subsiding spontaneously. Treatment: Analgesic and anti-inflammatory drugs.

REFERENCE

CHAUDHURI, R. N., and others (1951), *Lancet,* 1, 510.

BACK-POCKET SCIATICA ('Credit carditis' or the 'fat wallet syndrome')

Pain in sciatic distribution associated with an overfilled back pocket.

REFERENCE

GOULD, N. (1974), *New England Journal of Medicine,* 290, 633.

BEHÇET'S SYNDROME

A syndrome of unknown aetiology characterized by the triad of oral ulceration, genital ulceration, and iritis.

Incidence
Arthritis occurs in 60 per cent of cases.
M. 2 : 1.
Peak age of onset 20–40.
F.H. in 30 per cent.

Joints affected
Polyarticular.
Knees commonest (75 per cent).
Ankles often.
Occasionally elbows, wrists, small joints of hands, or feet. Neck, shoulders, hips uncommon. Symmetrical or asymmetrical. 10 per cent monarticular. Rarely migratory.

Symptoms
Insidious onset of pain and swelling.
Morning stiffness common.

Signs
Swelling, warmth, and effusion.

Course
Arthritis is chronic or episodic. Other manifestations are episodic, sometimes with remissions lasting many years. Attacks vary from a crop of ulcers with no systemic features to an acute severe febrile illness with polyarthritis and visceral manifestations. Neurological involvement may be fatal.

Associations
1. Mouth ulcers (100 per cent).
2. Genital ulcers (75 per cent).
3. Iritis (75 per cent).
4. Skin lesions (erythema nodosum, sepsis, or ulceration) (65 per cent).
5. Venous thrombosis (25 per cent).
6. Neurological manifestations (10 per cent): headache, confusion, coma, psychosis, cranial nerve palsies, fits, paralysis, cerebellar or spinal cord involvement, meningitis, or papilloedema.
   C.S.F. may show raised protein or slight increase in polymorphs and mononuclear cells.
7. Gastro-intestinal manifestations (50 per cent): diarrhoea, abdominal pain, nausea, flatulence, anorexia.

XR
Normal.

Laboratory
Raised E.S.R.
Leucocytosis (50 per cent).
Hyperglobulinaemia.
Joint fluid: inflammatory. Polymorph leucocytosis.
Latex test negative.

Treatment
Analgesic and anti-inflammatory drugs.
Steroids unhelpful.

REFERENCES

MASON, R. M., and BARNES, C. G. (1969), *Annals of the Rheumatic Diseases*, **28**, 95.
OSHIMA, Y., and others (1963), *Annals of the Rheumatic Diseases*, **22**, 36.

STRACHAN, R. W., and WIGZELL, F. W. (1963), *Annals of the Rheumatic Diseases*, **22**, 26.

BLASTOMYCOSIS

Systemic fungal infection caused by *Blastomyces dermatitidis*. Infection is usually manifest as a bronchopneumonia with purulent blood-stained sputum; metastatic lesions affect the skin and sometimes bones, joints, brain, and meninges. The disease occurs in North America and Southern Africa. Arthritis may be due to direct infection of the joint or extension from local osteomyelitis.

Incidence

M. = F.
Any age.
15 per cent have arthritis; 5 per cent present with joint pain.
Occurs at any time in the course of the disease.

Joints affected

Knee, ankle, wrist, or elbow commonest.
Occasionally small joints of hands or feet, hips, or shoulders.
Usually monarticular.

Symptoms

Acute onset of joint pain and swelling.

Signs

Effusion and soft-tissue swelling; sometimes warmth and erythema.

Course

Chronic with remissions and relapses.
Eventually fatal if untreated.

Associations

1. Pulmonary lesions are present in most cases; 50 per cent have productive cough or pleuritic chest pain. Fifty per cent have only changes on CXR: pleural effusion, bronchopneumonia, infiltration, consolidation with or without cavitation, miliary mottling, or hilar lymphadeno-pathy.
2. Skin and mucous membrane lesions in 50 per cent: chronic verrucous granulomata with surface micro-abscesses, spreading outwards and healing centrally, with considerable scarring. Discharging sinuses may be associated with underlying bone disease.
3. Lymphadenopathy (50 per cent). Splenomegaly occasionally.
4. Wasting and low-grade pyrexia.
5. Vertebral lesions may cause paraparesis.

XR

Normal if joint only affected; look for local osteomyelitis.

Laboratory

Microscopy of sputum, smears from skin lesions, synovial fluid, or biopsy material shows yeast cells of *B. dermatitidis*. Confirm by culture on Sabouraud's medium.
Skin tests and serology are of little value.
Synovial fluid: purulent.
Anaemia, raised E.S.R.
Slight polymorph leucocytosis.

Treatment

Amphotericin B (*see* p. 35).
Consider surgery, especially decompression for vertebral lesions.

Variant

Erythema nodosum (*see* p. 31).

REFERENCE

SANDERS, L. L. (1967), *Arthritis and Rheumatism*, **10**, 91.

BRUCELLOSIS

Infection with one of three *Brucella* organisms: *B. melitensis* from goats or sheep, *B. abortus* from cows, or *B. suis* from pigs. In Great Britain the disease is acquired from cows either by contact with infected animals or products of conception or by drinking raw milk or cream.

Incidence

M. 2 : 1.

Any age; commonest 20–40.

B. melitensis is the commonest cause of arthritis: 85 per cent have joint manifestations: arthralgia in 30 per cent, arthritis in 25 per cent, spondylitis in 50 per cent, sacro-iliitis in 35 per cent (unilateral in 60 per cent).

Arthritis less common with *B. suis* and *B. abortus* (arthralgia in 15 per cent, arthritis in 3 per cent, spondylitis in 3 per cent).

Farmers, butchers, veterinary surgeons, and country dwellers.

Joints affected

Arthralgia affects many joints and may be migratory.

Arthritis affects one to three joints; 50 per cent monarticular.

Knee, hip, and shoulder commonest.

Often sacro-iliac joint, wrist, ankle, or elbow.

Rarely small joints of hand or big toe.

Spondylitis affects lumbar spine in 70 per cent; any other area may be affected.

Symptoms

Pain in back and limbs common with febrile episodes.

Persistent localized pain in joints or spine suggests direct involvement.

Arthritis often preceded by general ill health, sweating, rigors, headaches, and weakness for several weeks or months.

Signs

Swelling, tenderness, warmth, and erythema usual.

Effusion often present.

Fever common (typically undulant but sometimes continuous or remittent).

Course

Usually transient, arthralgia lasting for a few days, arthritis for a few weeks, resolving completely without residua.

About 10 per cent have a more persistent arthritis with XR changes and may subsequently develop osteoarthritis, particularly of hip or knee.

Complications of spondylitis include pressure on nerve-roots and paravertebral, epidural, or psoas abscess.

Associations

1. Splenomegaly (25 per cent), hepatomegaly (5 per cent), lymphadenopathy (5 per cent).
2. Rash (various) in 10 per cent.
3. Bursitis, tendinitis, and nodules (rare).

XR

Peripheral joints usually normal. Porosis and destructive changes appear in 10 per cent.

Spine: disc narrowing with destruction of adjacent vertebra and new bone formation.

Large anterior spurs appear later in the spine. Osteophytes appear in peripheral joints.

Laboratory

W.B.C.: relative lymphocytosis and neutropenia in about 50 per cent.

Raised E.S.R. (85 per cent).

High or rising agglutination titre.

Isolation of *Brucella* from blood (20 per cent), joint fluid, bone-marrow, abscess or biopsy material should be repeatedly attempted.

Treatment

1. Septrin (trimethoprim + sulphamethoxazole) 2 g. daily for 4 weeks. Response is variable and relapse common; several courses of treatment are usually required.
2. Rest in acute stage, followed by gradual mobilization. Immobilization in a plaster cast required for cases of spondylitis with bone destruction.

REFERENCES

DALRYMPLE-CHAMPNEYS, W. (1960), *Brucella Infection and Undulant Fever in Man.* London: Oxford University Press.

ROTÉS-QUEROL, J. (1957), *Annals of the Rheumatic Diseases,* 16, 63.

ACUTE CALCIFIC PERIARTHRITIS

An acute inflammatory condition associated with the deposition of calcific material (hydroxy-apatite) in the periarticular soft tissues.

Incidence
M. = F.
Age 15 + ; typical onset at age 40.

Joints affected
Shoulder (50 per cent of attacks).
May affect big toe (resembling gout), fingers, hips, wrists, and knees.
Usually one joint only in each attack.

Symptoms
Sudden onset of pain, often very severe.

Signs
Affected joint may be red, hot, and tender in acute stage.

Course
Acute attacks, resolving completely without residua in 3 days to 3 weeks, but tending to recur at irregular intervals, months or years apart.

XR
Radio-opaque deposit adjacent to affected joint.

Laboratory
Raised E.S.R. and leucocytosis in acute stage.
Serum calcium normal.

Treatment
1. Indomethacin or phenylbutazone.
2. Injection of local anaesthetic and hydrocortisone into tender area.
3. Analgesics; morphine occasionally required in acute stage.
4. Surgery may be required to remove deposit, if chronic.

REFERENCE
SWANNELL, A. J., and others (1970), *Annals of the Rheumatic Diseases*, **29**, 380.

CALCIFICATION AND OSSIFICATION IN THE SPINE

Occurs in ankylosing spondylitis (*see* p. 7), ankylosing vertebral hyperostosis (*see* p. 8), ochronosis (*see* p. 86), psoriatic arthropathy—paravertebral ossification (*see* p. 105), pyrophosphate arthropathy (*see* p. 108), infective spondylitis, particularly brucellosis and syphilis (*see* p. 130), idiopathic hypoparathyroidism (*see* p. 56), hypophosphataemic spondylopathy (*see* p. 55), myositis ossificans (*see* p. 82), spondylo-epiphyseal dysplasia (*see* p. 18) and hereditary vascular and articular calcification (*see* p. 47).

REFERENCE
HART, F. D. (1968), *Lancet*, **1**, 740.

CALCIFICATION OF PERIARTICULAR SOFT TISSUES

Found in acute calcific periarthritis (*see above*), calcium phosphate deposition in patients after transplantation or on renal dialysis (*see* p. 112), neuropathic joints (*see* p. 83), some types of frozen shoulder (*see* p. 34), and tendinitis or bursitis at other sites, in hereditary vascular and articular calcification (*see* p. 47), scleroderma (*see* p. 121), and polymyositis (*see* p. 102), tumoral calcinosis (*see* p. 144), and myositis ossificans (*see* p. 82).

CAMPTODACTYLY

A slowly progressive painless flexion deformity of the little finger at the proximal interphalangeal joint, inherited as an autosomal dominant character. It is commoner in women (2 : 1) and develops during the first ten years of life. 70 per cent have bilateral involvement. No treatment is required. The condition must be distinguished from *Dupuytren's contracture* (*see* p. 26).

REFERENCE

SMITH, R. J., and KAPLAN, E. B. (1968), *Journal of Bone and Joint Surgery*, **50A**, 1187.

CARCINOID SYNDROME

A rare syndrome caused by the release of 5-hydroxytryptamine and other bioactive amines from liver metastases of a carcinoid tumour. The tumour arises from the argentaffin cells of the small intestine. Transient arthritis occurs rarely during the course of the disease, particularly causing symmetrical involvement of the interphalangeal joints of the fingers which are painful and swollen. Flexion contractures may develop. The usual features of the syndrome are attacks of facial flushing leading eventually to persistent erythema and telangiectasis of the face, weight-loss and cachexia, chronic diarrhoea, asthmatic attacks, a large irregular liver, and tricuspid or pulmonary valve disease. The diagnosis is confirmed by finding increased urinary 5-HIAA excretion. The condition is slowly progressive and patients often survive for many years.

REFERENCE

SJOERDSMA, A., and others (1956), *American Journal of Medicine*, **20**, 520.

CARCINOMA ARTHRITIS

A condition clinically resembling rheumatoid arthritis which occurs in patients with any type of malignant disease but particularly carcinoma of the bronchus, prostate, and breast, not due to metastases in bone or joint. This diagnosis is applicable to cases of arthritis which do not conform to other known patterns of arthritis associated with malignancy (*see* p. 71) and is probably not a single entity. Its importance lies in recognition of the underlying disease which is often treatable when arthritis appears.

Incidence
M. 2 : 1.
Peak age 50–65.
Onset typically about 1 year before but less commonly with or after manifestations of malignancy.

Joints affected
Knees, ankles, M.C.P. and M.T.P. joints commonest.
Often shoulders, elbows, wrists, hips, hands, and feet.
20 per cent monarticular.
50 per cent asymmetrical.

Symptoms
Sudden onset of joint pain, often severe; morning stiffness.

Signs
Joints may be warm, red, swollen, and tender in acute phase.

Course
Variable; usually remits with control of malignant disease. There may be acute episodes with complete or partial remissions or a chronic course progressing to severe disability.

Associations
Features of primary malignant disease.

XR
Usually normal.

Laboratory
E.S.R. often raised.
Latex test usually negative.
Synovial fluid: inflammatory.
No crystals.

Treatment
1. Control of associated malignant disease.
2. Anti-inflammatory drugs.

REFERENCE

MACKENZIE, A. H., and SCHERBEL, A. L. (1963), *Geriatrics*, **18**, 745.

CAT-SCRATCH FEVER

Infection with *Pasteurella multocida*. After a bite or scratch from a cat or dog, there is a local inflammatory reaction, which varies from minimal (sometimes not noticed by the patient) to severe with secondary infection, cellulitis, and abscess formation. This is associated with local lymph-node enlargement. The illness may persist for many weeks but eventually subsides. Septic arthritis is a rare complication which has been described in normal and rheumatoid joints. The diagnosis is confirmed by culture of synovial fluid; the condition responds rapidly to penicillin.

REFERENCE

BARTH, W. F., and others (1968), *Arthritis and Rheumatism*, **11**, 394.

CHIKUNGUNYA[1]

An epidemic arbor virus infection transmitted by the mosquito *Aedes aegypti*, found in Tanzania, Zambia, and Zaïre. After an incubation period of 3–12 days, there is a sudden onset of fever, joint pains, and later a rash. *O'nyong-nyong*[2] is a similar condition found in East Africa, also in epidemics due to an arbor virus but transmitted by the *Anopheles funestus* mosquito. It is distinguished by the association of lymphadenopathy; arthritis is similar in the two conditions.

Incidence

M. = F.
Any age; peak in children and young adults.
Arthritis is common.

Joints affected

Polyarticular.
Knees, elbows, wrists, fingers, and ankles commonest.
Large joints predominant.
Usually bilateral and symmetrical.

Symptoms

Sudden onset of severe pain, immobilizing the patient and preventing sleep.

Signs

Marked painful restriction of movement and tenderness.
Warmth and swelling rare.
Fever.

Course

Arthritis usually settles within a few weeks but rarely lasts for several months; eventually resolves without residua.
Fever lasts a few days but in chikungunya there may be a secondary rise after an afebrile period.

Associations

1. Itchy maculopapular rash (70 per cent) appears a few days after onset, on the trunk and limbs.
2. Headache, pain in the eye, and conjunctivitis especially in o'nyong-nyong.
3. Cervical lymph-node enlargement in o'nyong-nyong.

XR

Normal.

Laboratory

Leucopenia and relative lymphocytosis.

Treatment

1. Analgesics. Narcotics may be required.
2. Rest.

REFERENCES

[1] ROBINSON, M. C. (1955), *Transactions of the Royal Society of Tropical Medicine and Hygiene*, **49**, 28.

[2] SHORE, H. (1961), *Transactions of the Royal Society of Tropical Medicine and Hygiene*, **55**, 361.

CHONDROCALCINOSIS ARTICULARIS

The radiological appearance of linear calcification of articular cartilage in pyrophosphate arthropathy (*see* p. 108).

CHONDRODYSPLASIC RHEUMATISM

Arthritis as a feature of chondrodysplasia.

Multiple epiphyseal dysplasia is a condition characterized by abnormal development of the epiphyses of many bones, inherited as an autosomal dominant and manifest in childhood.

Spondylo-epiphyseal dysplasia is a similar condition in which there are also abnormalities of vertebral bodies. It may be transmitted as an autosomal dominant, manifest at birth, X-linked recessive, manifest in early childhood or autosomal recessive manifest in late childhood. Four types of arthritis occur:

1. Premature osteoarthritis is common, affecting particularly the hips.
2. Episodes of inflammatory polyarthritis occur and may affect the hands and feet with a bilateral symmetrical distribution resembling rheumatoid arthritis.
3. Acute pyrophosphate arthropathy and chrondrocalcinosis (*see* p. 108).
4. Spinal lesions with fusion of vertebrae which may resemble ankylosing spondylitis (*see* p. 7) or ochronosis (*see* p. 86).

Incidence

Rare.
M. = F. (except X-linked recessive which affects M only).
Any age but typically young adults.

Joints affected

There is involvement of epiphyses of hips, hands, shoulders, knees, and ankles. Osteoarthritis affects hips, knees, and ankles. Inflammatory polyarthritis affects multiple joints, including small joints of hands and feet.
Bilateral and symmetrical.

Symptoms

Pain, swelling, stiffness, restriction of movement, and difficulty in walking.

Signs

In acute episodes joints are red, warm, tender, and swollen with effusions. Late stage resembles osteoarthritis.

Course

Acute episodes may last for a few months. In severe cases, flexion deformities develop with progressive restriction of movement and eventually ankylosis.

Associations

Slight reduction in height especially in cases with spinal involvement.
Mental state and life expectancy normal.

XR

1. Late appearance and irregular ossification of epiphyses. Fragmentation of epiphyses may resemble osteochondritis dissecans. Multiple epiphyses involved throughout the body. This leads to flattened deformed articular surfaces, on which the changes of osteoarthritis are superimposed with loss of joint space, etc.
2. Cysts of variable size in the subchondral bone, particularly in the heads of metacarpals, phalanges, hips, and shoulders.
3. Osteochondral loose bodies.
4. Chondrocalcinosis.
5. Vertebral bodies are flat and wide—usually dorsolumbar spine.
6. Bony fusion of vertebrae—usually one but sometimes several adjacent discs involved. Sacro-iliac joints normal.

Laboratory

No metabolic abnormalities.
E.S.R. normal.
Latex test negative.
Synovial biopsy shows no evidence of synovitis.
Joint fluid may contain pyrophosphate crystals.

Treatment

Symptomatic—analgesic and anti-inflammatory drugs. Joint replacement may be required for advanced osteoarthritis.

REFERENCE

Kahn, M. F. (1970), *Annales de Médicine*, **121**, 1039.

CHYLOUS ARTHRITIS

Arthritis due to the presence of chyle within a joint. This is caused by lymphatic obstruction in filariasis, a nematode worm infestation which is endemic in India, tropical Asia and Africa, the West Indies, and South America. The worm is transmitted by mosquitoes. Infestation causes filarial fever (attacks of fever, lymphadenopathy, and sometimes urticaria), later chronic lymphadenopathy, and eventually lymphatic obstruction and elephantiasis.

Incidence
M. 2 : 1.
Any age, peak 20–40.

Joints affected
Knee.
Usually unilateral.

Symptoms
Sudden onset of pain and swelling.

Signs
In the acute stage, the joint is hot, tender, swollen with effusion, and marked limitation of movement.
Fever is usual.
Synovial thickening in the chronic stage.

Course
Acute attack subsides in 1–2 weeks. Attacks recur at irregular intervals but are milder than the initial episode.
Eventually arthritis may become chronic.

Associations
1. Large, tender, inguinal lymph-nodes are usually palpable.
2. Other evidence of lymphatic obstruction is only occasionally present, e.g., elephantiasis of a limb, or hydrocoele.

XR
Normal.
Lymphangiogram shows obstruction and varicosity of lymphatics.

Laboratory
W.B.C. normal or slightly raised.
Blood smear taken at midnight shows microfilariae in 30 per cent. Filarial complement-fixation test or skin test positive but non-specific.
Synovial fluid: thin, creamy-yellow fluid, resembling pus but sterile on culture. High lipid content (greater than blood level).
Lymph-node biopsy contra-indicated.

Treatment
1. Rest; analgesics; aspiration of fluid.
2. Diethylcarbamazine eliminates the worms.

REFERENCE

DAS, G. C., and SEN, S. B. (1968), *British Medical Journal*, 2, 27.

CIRRHOSIS OF THE LIVER

This is not usually associated with arthritis. However, a polyarthritis, particularly occurring in women, has been described in alcoholic cirrhosis. This affects shoulders, elbows, and knees most commonly, and is bilateral and symmetrical. There is pain and stiffness, sometimes with morning stiffness. Examination reveals soft-tissue swelling, tenderness, and small effusions. The condition is mild but chronic with relapses and remissions. XR are usually normal. Arthralgia has been reported in alcoholic and post-necrotic cirrhosis, again particularly in women. Bone changes resembling those found in familial hypercholesterolaemia have been described in biliary cirrhosis. Osteomalacia and secondary hyperparathyroidism (*see* p. 54) may also occur in this condition. The arthritis of chronic active hepatitis (juvenile cirrhosis), Wilson's disease, and haemochromatosis are described separately.

Polyarthralgia or polyarthritis is rarely associated with primary biliary cirrhosis. Joint involvement is bilateral and symmetrical with hands and knees the commonest sites. Arthritis is not progressive and may be episodic. The latex test is positive in 25 per cent of patients with primary biliary cirrhosis and may be misleading.

REFERENCES

ANSELL, B. M., and BYWATERS, E. G. L. (1957), *Annals of the Rheumatic Diseases*, 16, 503.
PACHAS, W. N., and PINALS, R. S. (1967), *Arthritis and Rheumatism*, 10, 343.

WILLCOX, R. G., and ISSELBACHER, K. J. (1961) *American Journal of Medicine*, 30, 185.
CHILD, D. L., and others (1977), *British Medical Journal*, 2, 557.

CLUTTON'S JOINTS

Bilateral hydrarthrosis of the knees associated with congenital syphilis. The condition is easily mistaken for Still's disease (*see* p. 62).

Incidence
M. = F.
Age 8–15 (rarely up to age 35).
About 10 per cent of congenital syphilitics have Clutton's joints.

Joints affected
Both knees but asymmetrical. One may precede the other by several years.
Rarely ankles or elbows.
Rarely unilateral.

Symptoms
Insidious onset of stiffness and swelling.
Pain often mild or absent.

Signs
Effusion.
Tenderness, limitation of movement, and warmth occasionally.
Fever common.

Course
Complete recovery in 3–12 months without residua.
Rarely lasts for several years.

Associations
Bilateral interstitial keratitis (40 per cent) and other stigmata of congenital syphilis, e.g., Hutchinson's teeth, nerve deafness, periostitis of tibia, typical facies.

XR
Normal.

Laboratory
Raised E.S.R.
Positive serological tests for syphilis.
Synovial fluid: inflammatory with polymorph leucocytosis.
Synovial biopsy: synovial proliferation, round-cell infiltration, and sometimes gummata.

Treatment
1. Penicillin should be given but does not influence the course of the arthritis.
2. Aspiration of fluid and injection of hydrocortisone for relief of symptoms.
3. Anti-inflammatory drugs have little effect.

REFERENCES

ARGEN, R. J., and DIXON, A. ST. J. (1963), *Arthritis and Rheumatism*, 6, 341.

CLUTTON, H. H. (1886), *Lancet*, 1, 391.

COCCIDIOIDOMYCOSIS

Dust-borne infection with the fungus *Coccidioides immitis*, endemic in the south-western part of the U.S.A. Infection may be subclinical or manifest as an influenza-like illness with pleuritic chest pain and patchy infiltration on chest X-ray (primary pulmonary coccidioidomycosis). Rarely the fungus becomes disseminated. Arthritis is of two types:

1. Arthritis occurs in about 5 per cent of cases of primary pulmonary coccidioidomycosis (desert rheumatism) associated with erythema nodosum, and less commonly erythema multiforme. Joint involvement has the characteristics of arthritis associated with erythema nodosum (*see* p. 31) affecting the knees and ankles particularly, and is associated with fever.

2. Arthritis occurs in about 10 per cent of cases of disseminated coccidioidomycosis.

Incidence

M. = F.
Any age, peak 25–55.
Particularly occurs in those who work with soil.

Joints affected

Knee commonest; any other joint or spine may be affected.
Affects one to three joints.
Usually monarticular.

Symptoms

Pain and swelling.

Signs

Swelling—large effusion and synovial thickening.
Limitation of movement.
Sometimes warm and red.

Course

Chronic. Progresses slowly to joint destruction.

Associations

1. Granulomatous or ulcerative skin lesions.
2. Lymphadenopathy.
3. Rarely meningitis.

XR

Early: normal.
Later: erosions, narrowing of joint space, irregularity of joint surface.

Laboratory

Coccidioidin skin-test (positive in 80 per cent). Complement-fixation test (positive in 60 per cent). Culture of the organism from synovial biopsy confirms. Synovial fluid often sterile. Synovial biopsy: granulomatous changes with marked proliferation and pannus formation.

Treatment

Amphotericin B.
Synovectomy often useful.

REFERENCE

POLLOCK, S. F., and others (1967), *Journal of Bone and Joint Surgery*, 49A. 1397.

COMPRESSION NEUROPATHIES

Compression or entrapment of nerves leads to a series of syndromes, the features of which depend on the nerve involved. Nerve compression syndromes cause pain which may be mistakenly attributed to arthritis; they also complicate arthritis and unless recognized are unlikely to be appropriately treated.

Features in common:
1. Pain worst at night with paraesthesiae in the distribution of the compressed nerve.
2. Pain may be felt proximal as well as distal to the site of compression but paraesthesiae only distally.
3. In the early stages there are symptoms only. Later there may be sensory impairment, hyperaesthesia, or hyperalgesia in the area supplied by the compressed nerve. Motor weakness and wasting are unusual, late and often irreversible.
4. Nerve conduction studies will demonstrate the site of compression.
5. Injection with hydrocortisone relieves symptoms at least temporarily and surgical decompression permanently.

Causes include:
1. Space-occupying lesions, ganglion, lipoma, etc.
2. Tenosynovitis of adjacent tendons.
3. Arthritis of adjacent joints, particularly rheumatoid arthritis.
4. Fractures of adjacent bones.
5. Direct injuries.
6. Conditions causing soft-tissue swelling. *See also* carpal tunnel and other individual syndromes. Many cases are idiopathic.

UPPER LIMB

Carpal tunnel syndrome: Compression of the median nerve in the carpal tunnel giving rise to pain in the wrist and hand, sometimes radiating upwards as far as the shoulder ('brachial neuritis') worst at night, associated with numbness and paraesthesia in the lateral $3\frac{1}{2}$ fingers and hand. Rarely there is thenar wasting. This is usually idiopathic, occurring particularly in the dominant hand of females (3 : 1) over the age of 40. It is bilateral in 50 per cent but is then worse in the dominant hand. When unilateral it affects the right hand about twice as often as the left. The syndrome is secondary in about 20 per cent of cases to *local conditions*, trauma (e.g., Colles fracture), tenosynovitis, ganglion, and lipoma or *generalized conditions*, hypothyroidism, acromegaly, pregnancy, amyloidosis, multiple myeloma and rheumatoid arthritis, or any other inflammatory arthropathy affecting the wrists. In these generalized conditions, symptoms are usually bilateral. Local steroid injection or immobilization in a splint will often be successful; if not, surgical division of the flexor retinaculum should be advised.

Pronator syndrome: Compression of the median nerve by pronator teres or fibrous arch of origin of flexor digitorum sublimis. Affects the dominant limb of men engaged in repetitive pronation. Symptoms similar to carpal tunnel syndrome but aggravated by use and not worse at night. Conduction studies show delay at forearm level. Decompression relieves symptoms.

Ulnar tunnel syndrome: Compression of the ulnar nerve in the ulnar tunnel causing pain and paraesthesiae on the medial side of the hand, impaired sensation in the medial $1\frac{1}{2}$ fingers, and weakness of the small muscles of the hand. Involvement of the deep branch causes wasting without sensory loss and is usually due to a ganglion. Excision of the volar carpal ligament relieves symptoms.

Ulnar nerve compression at the elbow caused by the fibrous arch of origin of flexor carpi ulnaris or less commonly condylar fracture, arthritis of the elbow, ganglion or hypermobility of the nerve, leads to pain in the hand which may radiate up the forearm with impaired sensation in the medial $1\frac{1}{2}$ fingers and palm and sometimes wasting of the small muscles of the hand. Division of the fibrous arch is usually sufficient treatment but anterior transposition of the ulnar nerve may occasionally be required.

Posterior interosseous nerve compression occurs at the fibrous origin of extensor carpi radialis brevis or between the two layers of supinator. It causes pain over the lateral epicondyle of the elbow and tenderness of the extensor origin, clinical features indistinguishable from those of tennis elbow. There may be weakness of the extensors of wrist and fingers. This diagnosis should be considered if a tennis elbow fails to respond to local injection.

Suprascapular nerve compression at the suprascapular notch causes pain in the shoulder and may be mistaken for frozen shoulder.

COMPRESSION NEUROPATHIES (*continued*)

LOWER LIMB

Tarsal tunnel syndrome: Compression of the posterior tibial nerve by the flexor retinaculum (lancinate ligament) which forms the tarsal tunnel between the medial malleolus and the calcaneum. There is burning pain with paraesthesiae in the toes and sole of foot, worse at night, relieved by movement or hanging the limb out of bed. The pain may radiate up the leg in sciatic distribution and be mistaken for sciatica. Symptoms of sensory loss may be confined to the territory of one of the divisions of the nerve, the medial plantar nerve supplying the medial $3\frac{1}{2}$ toes and sole, the lateral plantar nerve supplying the lateral $1\frac{1}{2}$ toes and sole, and the calcaneal nerve supplying the heel. Local swelling in the region of the tarsal tunnel and reproduction of symptoms by local pressure may provide clues to the correct diagnosis. Weakness of toe flexion is rare. Local steroid injection is helpful but surgical decompression may be required.

Common peroneal nerve compression occurs as the nerve winds round the neck of the fibula and may be caused by a plaster cast, tight boots, or direct trauma as well as the usual causes of compression. It may also be caused by inversion injuries to the ankle and is an important and often unsuspected cause of persistent disability after such an injury. There is pain in the lateral surface of the leg, ankle, and foot sometimes with sciatic radiation, often with nocturnal cramps and complaints of coldness of the leg. Impairment of sensation over the distal lateral surface of the leg and dorsum of foot often with striking weakness and instability of the ankles are characteristic. Shoes with a lateral sole wedge and analgesics may help. If operation is required it should include division of the fibrous origin of peroneus longus which may contribute to the compression.

Meralgia paraesthetica: Compression of the lateral femoral cutaneous nerve at the inguinal ligament or iliacus fascia causing burning pain, numbness, paraesthesiae, and hyperalgesia of the lateral border of the thigh. Local injection of prednisolone helps and operation is seldom required.

Ilio-inguinal nerve compression and **Obturator nerve compression** may cause pain in the groin which may be mistaken for hip pain. Symptoms may be aggravated by standing or hip movement. There is sensory loss below the inguinal ligament and on the inner side of the thigh. The symptoms of **Sciatic nerve compression** are well known to anyone who has 'sat on the nerve' and found that the leg has 'gone to sleep'. **Saphenous nerve compression** at the lower end of Hunter's canal causes pain in the medial side of the knee, radiating down the leg.

REFERENCE

KOPELL, H. P., and THOMPSON, W. A. L. (1963), *Peripheral Entrapment Neuropathies*. Baltimore: Williams & Wilkins.

CUTANEOUS POLYARTERITIS NODOSA

A rare condition which differs from polyarteritis nodosa in affecting only or predominantly the skin and having a good prognosis. Skin changes include painful nodules, ulceration and localized livedo reticularis, usually affecting the lower legs. About half of such cases have arthralgia and less often there is a chronic non-destructive polyarthritis resembling seronegative rheumatoid arthritis. It affects one or a few sites, bilateral and symmetrical. Joints are swollen and there may be effusions. It pursues a chronic prolonged course but the prognosis is good and life-threatening complications of polyarteritis nodosa do not occur. E.S.R. is raised. Synovial fluid is inflammatory with W.B.C. up to $20,000 \times 10^9$/dl., mainly polymorphs. The diagnosis can only be confirmed by skin biopsy. XR is usually normal and erosions do not occur. Treatment: Non-steroidal anti-inflammatory drugs.

REFERENCES

DIAZ-PEREZ, J. L., and WINKLEMANN, R. K. (1974), *Archives of Dermatology*, **110**, 407.

SMUCKLER, N. M., and SCHUMACHER, H. R. (1976), *Arthritis and Rheumatism*, **20**, 114.

DEEP VEIN THROMBOSIS

Most deep vein thromboses occurring in patients with arthritis are really due to joint rupture.[1] It is particularly common in rheumatoid arthritis but may occur in osteoarthritis and any other condition which causes a knee effusion. There is a sudden onset of pain in the calf associated with swelling of the ankle. There is calf tenderness and Homan's sign is positive. The knee often improves after rupture and the patient may forget about it when recounting his story. The diagnosis is swiftly confirmed by injection of radio-opaque contrast into the joint. XR shows contrast material tracking into the calf. Treatment is with rest and injection of prednisolone into the knee. Patients with true deep vein thrombosis may be unable to extend the knee of the affected leg and this may cause confusion.[2]

REFERENCES

[1]Dixon, A. St. J., and Grant, C. (1964), *Lancet*, **1**, 742.

[2]Corrigan, T. P., and Strachan, C. J. L. (1973), *British Medical Journal*, **4**, 296.

DENGUE

An arbor virus infection transmitted from monkey to man by the mosquito (*Aedes aegypti*). It occurs in epidemics widespread in tropical Asia, India, Africa, and South America. After an incubation period of 4–14 days, there is a sudden onset of fever which lasts for about a week; there may be an afebrile period followed by a secondary rise in temperature (saddleback fever). Joint pain is common and occurs with the onset of fever. It is characteristically very severe and may affect one or many joints. Movement is restricted by pain, and there is tenderness over tendons and muscle insertions. Joints are not hot or swollen. Joint pain usually continues for a few days but occasionally for weeks. An itchy rash appears on the fourth day which is maculopapular or scarlatiniform. XR are normal. Leucopenia with relative lymphocytosis is characteristic; the diagnosis can be confirmed in retrospect by demonstrating a rise in antibody titre. Treatment: Salicylates; stronger analgesics required if pain is severe.

REFERENCE

Manson-Bahr, P. H. (1954), *Manson's Tropical Diseases*, London: Cassell.

DRUG-INDUCED ARTHRALGIA AND ARTHRITIS

Aches and pains in joints and muscles may on occasion be caused, or precipitated, by drugs.

1. Acute gout may be precipitated by oral diuretics, an exception being triamterene, by intramuscular injections of mersalyl, and by uricosuric drugs (e.g., probenecid, sulphinpyrazone). Allopurinol may also have the same effect early in the course of treatment. Radioactive phosphorus in the treatment of primary polycythaemia and cytotoxic drugs in the therapy of chronic leukaemia and other malignant disorders may precipitate acute episodes, as may the antituberculous drug pyrazinamide, some antihypertensive drugs (pempidine, mecamylamine), and large doses of nicotinic acid. Small doses of aspirin antagonize the action of uricosuric drugs, while large doses (5 g. or more daily) are themselves uricosuric.

2. Rheumatoid arthritis may be exacerbated by iron-dextran when given by the total-dose method, and arthralgia may be experienced in non-rheumatoids. Too rapid withdrawal, or sudden stopping, of corticosteroid therapy may precipitate a diffuse arteritis or neuropathy in rheumatoid arthritis.

3. Systemic lupus erythematosus may be exacerbated or precipitated by a large number of drugs, the commonest being penicillin and sulphonamides, but oral contraceptives may, rarely, be responsible.

4. The lupus-like hydrallazine syndrome is described on p. 26. It may be caused by a large variety of drugs, the commonest being procaine amide.

5. Polyarteritis nodosa may also be precipitated or exacerbated by the sulphonamides, penicillin, and a number of other drugs.

6. The serum-sickness type of reaction may occur with a variety of drugs, the commonest being the penicillins and barbiturates (p. 124).

DRUG-INDUCED ARTHRALGIA AND ARTHRITIS (*continued*)

7. Pains, aches, and odd sensations may occur early in drug-induced polyneuropathy (e.g., nitrofurantoin), myopathy (e.g., triamcinolone, and rarely digitalis and some antihypertensive drugs), or Parkinsonism (e.g., chlorpromazine). Aching in the legs and back may be early symptoms of retroperitoneal fibroplasia due to methysergide. A variety of muscle aches have been reported with the oral contraceptives. Suxamethonium may cause severe muscle pain after it has been given to induce muscle relaxation for surgery.

8. Fluid retention may cause muscle aches, but rarely to a severe degree. This has been reported with oral contraceptives, oestrogens, androgens, the corticosteroids and corticotrophins, reserpine, and carbenoxolone.

9. Sodium depletion may cause muscle aches and cramps with over-enthusiastic diuretic and spironolactone therapy.

10. Aching muscles may be due to hypokalaemia caused by over-use of diuretics, carbenoxolone and liquorice extracts, corticosteroids and corticotrophins, purges, or, very rarely, chlorpromazine and sodium aminosalicylate.

11. Magnesium depletion due to prolonged purgation rarely causes myalgia and muscle cramps.

12. Crush fractures in osteoporotic vertebrae may cause considerable discomfort, the corticosteroids often being responsible. Less severe aching in the spine may also be due to osteomalacia induced by prolonged use of laxatives or aluminium hydroxide.

13. The barbiturates may rarely cause arthralgia accompanied by contractures, the so-called 'rheumatisme barbiturique'.

14. The shoulder–hand syndrome has been attributed to isoniazid and to barbiturate therapy.

15. Acute haemarthrosis may occur with anticoagulant overdosage. The affected joint is swollen, red and very tender, but settles within a few days.

16. High-dose steroid therapy causes avascular necrosis (*see* p. 10). Arthralgia may be associated with chronic steroid overdosage and has been described as steroid pseudorheumatism. There is also an increased liability to develop infections including septic arthritis (*see* p. 123) in patients on steroids.

17. Repeated intra-articular injections of antibiotics cause post-infectious synovitis (*see* p. 123). Repeated intra-articular steroid injections may cause destructive changes in the joint; crystalline steroid preparations may cause arthritis.

18. A condition resembling avascular necrosis of the shoulder has been described in bismuth poisoning.[2]

Moral: when in doubt in an unexplained cause of arthralgia or arthritis, try stopping any non-essential drugs the patient may be taking.

REFERENCES

[1] *Adverse Drug Reaction Bulletin* (1971), **30**, 88.

[2] Buge, A., and others (1975), *Revue du Rhumatisme* **42**, 721.

DRUG-INDUCED S.L.E. (the Hydrallazine Syndrome)

A condition resembling systemic lupus erythematosus but induced by procainamide, hydrallazine, phenytoin and related compounds, isoniazid, oral contraceptives, penicillin, sulphonamides, tetracycline, streptomycin, griseofulvin, phenylbutazone, penicillamine, thiouracils, reserpine, and methyldopa. It is suggested that patients with this condition have a hereditary 'lupus diathesis' which is made manifest only when the drug is given.

Incidence

M. = F.
Age 40+.
Arthralgia or arthritis in 70 per cent; presenting feature in 60 per cent.
Affects up to 30 per cent of patients on procainamide, 10 per cent on hydrallazine, others rare. Not related to dosage. Onset 2 weeks to 6 years after start of therapy.

Joints affected

Polyarticular, as in S.L.E.
P.I.P. joints of hands commonest.
Bilateral and symmetrical.
Often migratory.

Symptoms

Joint pain.
Malaise.

Signs

Often none.
Typically soft-tissue swelling only.
Fever in 40 per cent.

Course

Disappears rapidly on stopping the causative drug, though serological abnormalities may persist for many years.

Associations

1. Pleurisy (50 per cent).
2. Other systemic features less common than with S.L.E.: rashes (10 per cent), pericarditis (15 per cent), hepatomegaly (25 per cent), splenomegaly (10 per cent), and lymphadenopathy (5 per cent).
3. Renal manifestations: proteinuria occurs rarely but never renal failure. Fits and other C.N.S. manifestations do not occur.

XR

Normal.

Laboratory

L.E. cells (90 per cent) and A.N.F. (always) positive.
No anti-DNA antibodies.
E.S.R. often raised.
Leucopenia (20 per cent).

Treatment

Stop the drug.
Steroids may be given for symptomatic relief but are not necessary.

REFERENCES

ALARCON-SEGOVIA, D. (1969), *Proceedings of Staff Meetings of the Mayo Clinic*, **44**, 664.
HARPEY, J. P. (1973), *Adverse Drug Reaction Bulletin*, No. 43, p. 140.

SHELDON, P. J. H. S., and WILLIAMS, W. R. (1970), *Annals of the Rheumatic Diseases*, **29**, 236.

DUPUYTREN'S CONTRACTURE

A common condition in which progressive fibrosis of the palmar fascia causes painless flexion contractures of the fingers. It affects the white race only, particularly men (8 : 1) and begins after age 25. It is occasionally familial (probably inherited as an autosomal dominant) and there is a high incidence in patients with liver disease, especially alcoholic, and epilepsy. The ring finger is affected first and most severely (65 per cent), then the little finger (55 per cent) and the middle finger (25 per cent) and, rarely, the index finger (5 per cent) or thumb (3 per cent). Puckering of the skin of the palm is characteristic with palpable thickening of and sometimes nodules in the palmar fascia. It is usually bilateral. Unusual associations include Peyronie's and knuckle pads (*see* p. 64). Treatment: Selective fasciectomy.

DUPUYTREN'S CONTRACTURE (*continued*)

Other causes of flexion contractures of the fingers to be excluded:
1. Diseases of the joints and/or tendons:
   Rheumatoid arthritis (*see* p. 114).
   Scleroderma (*see* p. 121).
   Late stage of shoulder–hand syndrome (*see* p. 125).
   Still's disease (*see* p. 61).
   Psoriatic arthropathy (*see* p. 105).
   Some rare arthropathies (*see* individual descriptions).
2. Muscle weakness due to neurological lesions or immobilization.
3. Scarring following trauma, burns, or infection.
4. Volkmann's ischaemic contracture.
5. Soft-tissue tumours in the palm.
6. Malformation syndromes:[2]
   Marfan's syndrome.
   Congenital contractural arachnodactyly.
   Arthrogryposis (*see* p. 9).
   Melorheostosis (*see* p. 72).
   Trisomy 13.
   Craniocarpotarsal syndrome.
   Diastrophic dwarfism.
   Kushokwim syndrome.
7. Camptodactyly (*see* p. 16).
8. Leri's pleonosteosis (*see* p. 66).

REFERENCES

[1] VILJANTO, J. A. (1973), *Seminars in Arthritis and Rheumatism*, 3, 155.
[2] WYNNE-DAVIES, R. (1973), *Hereditable Disorders in Orthopedic Practice*. Oxford: Blackwell.

DYSPROTEINAEMIC ARTHROPATHY

Arthralgia is common in a number of disorders in which there are abnormalities of serum proteins. These include cryoglobulinaemias and paraproteinaemias such as myeloma. Joint involvement is polyarticular, bilateral and symmetrical. Many abnormal proteins have rheumatoid factor-like activity and a positive latex test may obscure the correct diagnosis.

REFERENCES

ZAWADZKI, Z. A., and BENEDEK, T. G. (1969), *Arthritis and Rheumatism*, 12, 555.
MELTZER, M., and others (1966), *American Journal of Medicine*, 40, 837.

ENTEROPATHIC SYNOVITIS

Arthritis associated with ulcerative colitis[1] or Crohn's disease.[2] Apart from enteropathic synovitis (described below) three other types of arthritis occur in these diseases.

1. *Ankylosing spondylitis*: 5 per cent of patients with either ulcerative colitis or Crohn's disease have ankylosing spondylitis (*see* p. 7). This affects women as commonly as men, is not related to the extent, severity, or localization of gut disease, often precedes the development of gut disease, and progresses despite surgery.
2. *Arthritis* associated with erythema nodosum (*see* p. 31).
3. *Pseudohypertrophic osteoarthropathy* (*see* p. 104).

Incidence

M. = F.
Peak age 25–55.
In ulcerative colitis 12 per cent develop arthritis; in Crohn's disease 20 per cent develop arthritis.
Arthritis usually occurs within the first few years of colitis and is more common in patients with extensive disease. In Crohn's disease it is more common in patients with small bowel involvement. In 10 per cent arthritis precedes gut manifestations.

Joints affected

Knee (70 per cent) and ankle (50 per cent) commonest.
Often elbows, wrists, or fingers.
Occasionally shoulders, hips, or feet.
Usually one to three joints in each attack.
Usually asymmetrical. May be migratory.

Symptoms

Sudden onset of pain and swelling, often associated with relapse of bowel disease.

Signs

Effusion.
Painful limitation of movement.
Occasionally erythema.

Course

Attacks last 1–2 months.
Most patients have only 1–3 attacks and each resolves completely.
Arthritis remits after colectomy in ulcerative colitis but surgery produces remission in only 35 per cent of cases of Crohn's disease.
Surgery has no effect on associated ankylosing spondylitis.

Associations

1. Abdominal pain, diarrhoea, rectal bleeding, constipation, weight loss, debility, fever.
2. Skin lesions: erythema nodosum, pyoderma gangrenosum (25 per cent).
3. Uveitis (20 per cent).
4. Buccal ulceration (30 per cent).
5. Perianal disease, fissure, or fistula (20 per cent).
6. Clubbing of the fingers (10 per cent).
7. In Crohn's disease there may be internal or external fistulae (25 per cent) or malabsorption (5 per cent).

Systemic complications are commoner with enteropathic synovitis in ulcerative colitis but not in Crohn's disease.

XR

Joints normal.
Sacro-iliitis in 20 per cent.
Ankylosing spondylitis in 5 per cent. Barium follow-through or enema to show intestinal disease.

Laboratory

Raised E.S.R.
Latex test negative.
Synovial fluid: inflammatory;
W.B.C. up to $40,000 \times 10^9/dl.$, predominantly neutrophils.

Treatment

1. Analgesic and anti-inflammatory drugs.
2. Appropriate treatment for gut disease.

REFERENCES

[1] WRIGHT, V., and WATKINSON, G. (1965), *British Medical Journal*, **2**, 670.

[2] HASLOCK, I. (1973), *Annals of the Rheumatic Diseases*, **32**, 479.

EOSINOPHILIC FASCIITIS

A skin condition characterized by thickening and induration of the skin, which may be accompanied by joint pain and stiffness. The condition is probably a variant of scleroderma but visceral changes and Raynaud's phenomenon are usually absent. The diagnosis is suggested by the finding of eosinophilia and confirmed by a full-thickness skin biopsy which shows thickening of subcutaneous fascia and infiltration with lymphocytes and plasma cells. Joints are involved in a bilateral symmetrical distribution. There may be arthralgia or occasionally synovitis. Skin changes are found on the arms, legs or trunk with sparing of the hands and face. Severe skin involvement may lead to joint contractures. The skin is brawny and hidebound. Hypergammaglobulinaemia is common but A.N.F. and rheumatoid factor are negative. The condition responds to corticosteroids and prognosis is good.

REFERENCES

RODNAN, G. P., and others (1975), *Arthritis and Rheumatism*, **18**, 422.

BENNETT, R. M., and others (1977), *Annals of Rheumatic Diseases*, **36**, 354.

EPIDEMIC AUSTRALIAN POLYARTHRITIS

Arthritis due to infection with an arbor virus, known as Ross River virus. It occurs only in Australia. After an incubation period of about 10 days, patients develop either a rash or joint pains. The illness is mild.

Incidence
M. = F.
Any age; peak in young adults.
65 per cent have joint pain.
Joint pain precedes the rash in 50 per cent by up to 1 week.

Joints affected
Polyarticular.
M.C.P. or P.I.P. joints of hands (50 per cent) and knees (50 per cent) commonest.
Occasionally feet, shoulders, ankles, and wrists.
Usually symmetrical.

Symptoms
Pain, often mild.
Stiffness.

Signs
Limitation of movement.
Swelling occasionally; warmth, erythema, and effusion rare.
Temperature usually normal.

Course
Arthritis resolves completely within 4 weeks, without residua.

Associations
1. Rash. Pink macules up to 10 mm. in diameter appear on the cheeks and spread to involve the rest of the body. They blanch on pressure and do not itch. They occasionally become papular, rarely vesicular, and fade in 2 days to 2 weeks.
2. Malaise, headache, backache, and painful lymphadenopathy occasionally.

XR
Normal.

Laboratory
W.B.C. normal.

Treatment
Salicylates.

REFERENCE

ANDERSON, S. G., and FRENCH, E. L. (1957), *Medical Journal of Australia*, **2**, 113.

ERYTHEMA INFECTIOSUM

An uncommon epidemic exanthem of presumed viral aetiology affecting predominantly children (80 per cent) under age 15, usually in the spring. After an incubation period of 5–14 days, an itchy rash develops, at first on the cheeks, and later on the hands and feet spreading proximally. The lesions are papular and coalesce to form a large erythematous area resembling erysipelas (the 'slapped-cheek' appearance); they have a tendency to appear and disappear rapidly.

Incidence
F. 2 : 1.
Arthritis in 70 per cent of adults and 10 per cent of children.
Synchronous with other manifestations.

Joints affected
Wrists and knees commonest.
Other large joints may be affected.

Symptoms
Joint pain and swelling.

Signs
Affected joints are usually swollen; rarely normal.
Fever in 20 per cent.

Course
Illness usually lasts 1–2 weeks but occasionally up to 3 months.
Arthritis resolves completely without residua.

Associations
1. Exanthem.
2. Sometimes dark-red macules on mucous membranes.
3. Malaise, headache, myalgia, and gastro-intestinal disturbance.

XR
Normal.

Laboratory
Leucocytosis with eosinophilia and lymphocytosis.
No diagnostic test; cultures sterile.

Treatment
Salicylates.

REFERENCES

AGER, E. A., and others (1966), *New England Journal of Medicine*, **275**, 1326.

ROOK, A. (1968), in *Textbook of Dermatology* (ed. ROOK, A., WILKINSON, D. S., and EBLING, F. J. G.). Oxford: Blackwell.

ERYTHEMA MULTIFORME

Polyarthritis is a rare complication, reported in only 1 of 81 cases reviewed. Arthritis occurs in association with erythema multiforme in histoplasmosis (*see* p. 50), coccidioidomycosis (*see* p. 22), and lymphogranuloma venereum (*see* p. 64).

REFERENCE

ASHBY, D. W., and LAZAR, T. (1951), *Lancet*, **1**, 1091.

ERYTHEMA NODOSUM

An acute self-limiting condition characterized by the development of crops of tender nodules in the skin of the lower leg. The nodules are at first bright red, later dark red, and fade like bruises. The condition occurs in: (1) *Sarcoidosis*, the commonest cause in Great Britain, accounting for about 35 per cent of cases. (2) *Various infections*, particularly after streptococcal infection and in primary tuberculosis; also blastomycosis, cat-scratch fever, coccidioidomycosis, histoplasmosis, leprosy (erythema nodosum leprosum, *see* p. 65), lymphogranuloma venereum, measles, and psittacosis. (3) *Ulcerative colitis* and *Crohn's disease*. (4) *Malignant disease*, particularly lymphoma and leukaemia. (5) *Drug sensitivities*, e.g., to sulphonamides. (6) *Behçet's syndrome* (*see* p. 12). (7) *Idiopathic*. In about 10 per cent of cases no cause is found.

Incidence

F. 5 : 1.
Any age, usually 20–60.
Arthritis occurs in 50 per cent of cases, often synchronous with skin lesions; may precede skin lesions by up to 4 weeks.

Joints affected

Knees (85 per cent) and ankles (75 per cent) commonest.
Often elbows, wrists, shoulders, M.C.P. and P.I.P. joints of hands.
Occasionally hips, spine, and feet.
Starts in one joint but spreads to affect many within a few days.
Usually symmetrical eventually (90 per cent).

Symptoms

Sudden onset of pain with or without swelling.
Morning stiffness common.

Signs

None or red, swollen, tender joints.
Small effusion occasionally.
Fever common.

Course

Arthritis subsides completely without residua in 6 months or less.
Skin lesions last up to 6 weeks but sometimes recur.

XR

Joints normal.
CXR shows hilar lymphadenopathy in 80 per cent of cases of sarcoidosis with erythema nodosum and arthritis.

Laboratory

Raised E.S.R.
Latex test occasionally positive.
Routine diagnostic tests required for causative conditions: full blood-count, throat swab, ASO titre, sputum for tuberculosis, Mantoux test.
Consider lymph-node biopsy, Kveim test, and biopsy of other organs, e.g., liver for sarcoidosis.

Treatment

1. Rest in acute stage.
2. Aspirin or other anti-inflammatory drugs.

REFERENCE

TRUELOVE, L. H. (1960), *Annals of the Rheumatic Diseases*, 19, 174.

FAMILIAL ARTHROPATHY WITH RASH, UVEITIS AND MENTAL RETARDATION

A very rare genetic disorder which presents in childhood and may resemble juvenile chronic arthritis (p. 61). Clinical features include a rash resembling that of Still's disease (p. 61), mental retardation, failure to thrive, lymphadenopathy, arthropathy and uveitis. It begins at birth, is polyarticular and progresses rapidly to joint contractures. XRs show severe disorganization of epiphyses. Laboratory: Anaemia and raised E.S.R.

REFERENCE

ANSELL, B. M., and others (1975), *Proceedings of the Royal Society of Medicine*, 68, 24.

FAMILIAL HISTIOCYTIC DERMATOARTHRITIS

A very rare disorder which resembles multicentric reticulohistiocytosis. It is inherited as an autosomal dominant and presents in childhood and adolescence. Features include a symmetrical destructive arthritis indistinguishable from that of multicentric reticulohistiocytosis, cutaneous and ocular lesions. Cutaneous nodules are found on the ears, face, hands or feet and flat plaques are palpable in the skin of the extremities. Ocular lesions include glaucoma, uveitis and cataract. Histology of the early nodule shows a granulomatous lesion with lymphocyte and plasma cell infiltration. Later it becomes less cellular and there are histiocytes, fibroblasts and collagen. The plaques show fibroblasts and collagen. The synovium shows only fibrous thickening.

REFERENCE

ZAYID, I., and FARRAJ, S. (1973), *American Journal of Medicine*, **54**, 793.

FAMILIAL MEDITERRANEAN FEVER

A condition affecting people of Mediterranean origin, mostly Sephardic Jews but also Armenians and Levantine Arabs, characterized by recurrent acute attacks of fever and arthritis. It is inherited as an autosomal recessive character. In addition to the arthritis described below.[1,2] 17 per cent have ankylosing spondylitis[3] (M. 5 : 2) and 30 per cent have bilateral sacro-iliitis on X-ray.

Incidence

M. 3 : 2.
Onset usually age 1–15, occasionally up to 40.
70 per cent have joint pain at some time.

Joints affected

One joint in each attack.
Knee commonest, also ankle, hip, shoulder, and elbow.
Hands and feet seldom affected.

Symptoms

Acute onset of pain of variable severity.
No morning stiffness. May be precipitated by exertion or trauma.

Signs

Severe attacks accompanied by local muscle spasm and tenderness.
Heat and redness usually absent.
Small effusion often.
Muscle wasting in prolonged attacks.

Course

Attacks recur at irregular intervals, days or years apart. There may be:
1. Transient arthralgia during a febrile episode.
2. Arthritis lasting up to 1 week.
3. Occasionally arthritis lasting for weeks or months.
Complete recovery follows without sequelae.

Associations

1. Attacks of fever with abdominal or chest pain.
2. Amyloidosis in about 30 per cent leading to renal failure and fatal in 5–10 years.

XR

Normal except in prolonged attacks when porosis and erosions may develop.
Complete resolution follows but degenerative changes may develop over the years.

Laboratory

E.S.R. normal or raised.
Leucocytosis may occur.

Treatment

Analgesics. Colchicine (0·5 mg. b.d. or t.d.s.) prevents attacks in most patients.[4]
Steroids ineffective.

REFERENCES

[1] EHRENFELD, E. N., and others (1961), *American Journal of Medicine*, **31**, 107.
[2] HELLER, H., and others (1966), *Arthritis and Rheumatism*, **9**, 1.
[3] DILSEN, N. A. (1973), *Excerpta Medica International Congress Series*, **299**, 364.
[4] *British Medical Journal* (1975), **3**, 60.

FARBER'S DISEASE (Disseminated Lipogranulomatosis)

A very rare type of mucopolysaccharidosis inherited as an autosomal recessive character. Pathologically there is infiltration of tissues with mucopolysaccharide and lipid material accompanied by a granulomatous reaction. Arthritis is a prominent feature.

Incidence

M. = F.

Onset in the first few months of life.

Joint manifestations

1. Red, swollen, tender joints. All joints are affected; bilateral and symmetrical.
2. Pigmented nodular swellings appear in the periarticular soft tissues.

Course

Arthritis progresses rapidly to ankylosis with flexion contractures causing complete immobility.

Death is usual before age 2 from respiratory infection.

Associations

1. Hoarse cry; stridor; respiratory difficulty.
2. Mental retardation and motor impairment.
3. Vomiting, diarrhoea, and feeding problems.
4. Abnormal appearance with coarse facies and macroglossia.

XR

Osteoporosis and erosion.

Laboratory

Increased urinary excretion of chondroitin sulphate B.

Treatment

Symptomatic.

REFERENCE

BIERMAN, S. M., and others (1966), *Arthritis and Rheumatism*, 9, 620.

FLUOROSIS

Prolonged ingestion of excessive fluoride in food or water leads in man to changes roughly resembling ankylosing spondylitis. Osteosclerosis with periosteal new bone formation, vertebral osteophyte formation and calcification of paravertebral ligaments resemble the changes of ankylosing spondylitis. But the classical radiological changes in the sacro-iliac joints are absent. The affected bones contain fluoride; serum alkaline phosphate levels are raised. The usual complaints are of stiffness of back and hips.[1] A diagnostic sign is mottled enamel of the second dentition. Occupational fluorosis may occur in factories where cryolite (sodium and aluminium fluoride) is powdered preparatory to the production of aluminium.[2]

REFERENCES

[1]SINGH, A., JOLLY, S. S., and BANSAL, B. C. (1961), *Lancet*, 1, 197.

[2]BOSWORTH, T. J., GREEN, H. H., and MURRAY, M. M. (1941), *Proceedings of the Royal Society of Medicine*, 34, 391.

FRANCOIS SYNDROME (Familial Dermochondrocorneal Dystrophy)

A very rare disorder inherited as an autosomal recessive and characterized by epiphyseal dysplasia leading to deformities of the hands and feet, skin nodules and corneal opacities. It begins in the first two years of life, affects the small joints of the hands and feet but no others and progresses to subluxation and fixed deformities by the age of 12. XR show aplastic and irregular epiphysis. The nodules are found on the dorsum of the hands and resemble xanthomata. They may ulcerate and discharge. Histologically they contain large cells with cytoplasmic vacuoles. Serum cholesterol is usually normal and there are no other laboratory abnormalities. There is no treatment.

REFERENCE

McKUSICK, V. A. (1972), *Hereditable Disorders of Connective Tissue*, 4th ed. St. Louis: Mosby.

FROZEN SHOULDER

General term for pain in the shoulder which arises from a number of different conditions, not always clinically distinguishable: (1) *Tendinitis* (supraspinatus, infraspinatus, subscapularis, long head of biceps). (2) *Subacromial bursitis*. (3) *Traumatic lesions of the rotator cuff*. (4) *Capsulitis*, a doubtful pathological entity. Any of these conditions may be accompanied by pain in the arm and hand, the shoulder–hand syndrome (*see* p. 125), and conditions which cause the shoulder–hand syndrome may cause frozen shoulder without symptoms in the arm and hand.

Incidence
Commoner in males.
Age 40+.

Joints affected
Shoulder.
Usually unilateral.

Symptoms
Pain, often worse at night.
May be precipitated by unusual exertion, e.g. home decorating.

Signs
Painful limitation of movement; painful arc (45–135° of abduction) with lesions of rotator cuff.
Local tenderness indicates the site of the lesion, e.g., over the supraspinatus, infraspinatus, or biceps tendon.

Course
Chronic; lasts up to 2 years, then recovers completely.
If shoulder is immobilized, restriction of movement may be permanent.

Associations
Features of shoulder–hand syndrome (*see* p. 125).

XR
Usually normal.
Rarely calcification in tendons.

Laboratory
Normal E.S.R. Otherwise unhelpful.

Treatment
1. Restore and maintain full mobility; physiotherapy, heat or cold sometimes useful.
2. Local steroid injection for relief of symptoms and as an aid to mobilizing a stiff joint. Choose the area of maximum tenderness.
3. Analgesics and anti-inflammatory drugs for relief of symptoms. Propionic acid derivatives most suitable.

REFERENCE

BOYLE, A. C. (1969), *British Medical Journal*, **3**, 283.

FUNGUS INFECTIONS

Arthritis occurs in fungal infections: (1) As a result of direct infection of the joint. (2) By direct extension from adjacent bone infection, or (3) In association with erythema nodosum or erythema multiforme. Fungus infections are endemic in certain parts of the world, but occur also in patients with depressed immunity, on steroids or immuno-suppressive drugs and with lymphoma, leukaemia or other malignancy, aplastic anaemia or sarcoidosis (opportunistic infection).

Arthritis is an important feature of:

Blastomycosis (see p. 13).   *Histoplasmosis (see* p. 49).
African histoplasmosis (see p. 3).   *Coccidioidomycosis (see* p. 21).

It is a rare feature of the following fungal infections:

Cryptococcosis (Torulosis). A dust-borne infection wih *Cryptococcus neoformans*, found throughout the world particularly as an opportunist. Inhalation of the fungus, which is present in dust and pigeon excreta, causes pneumonitis, often subclinical. Dissemination is rare. Monarticular involvement of knee, wrist, elbow, or sternoclavicular joint may result; the affected joint is painful and swollen with limitation of movement, effusion, and tenderness. X-ray shows well-defined osteolytic areas adjacent to the joint. The diagnosis is confirmed by culture of biopsy material from the joint.

Treatment: Amphotericin B (*see below*).

REFERENCE

GOSLING, H. R., and GILMER, W. S. (1956), *Journal of Bone and Joint Surgery*, **38A**, 660.

Aspergillosis. Infection with *Aspergillus fumigatus*, a fungus found throughout the world in decomposing vegetable matter, usually complicates either pre-existing lung disease (cavitating tuberculosis, bronchiectasis, or asthma) or occurs as an opportunistic infection. Disease is usually pulmonary or allergic, but rarely becomes disseminated. Arthritis of the wrist and spine has been reported, causing painful swelling and leading to marked bone destruction. The diagnosis is made by culturing synovial fluid or biopsy material from the joint.

Treatment: Amphotericin B (*see below*).

REFERENCE

SHAW, W., and WARTHEN, H. J. (1936), *Southern Medical Journal*, **29**, 1070.

Mycetoma (Madura Foot). Infection with a number of fungi which affects those who walk barefoot in tropical and subtropical areas. The area of the tarsometatarsal joints is affected. Nodules form which ulcerate and cause discharging sinuses. The condition is usually painless.

Treatment: Infection with actinomycotic fungi responds to prolonged treatment with sulphadiazine. Drainage, excision, and sometimes amputation are required for the mucormycotic type.

REFERENCE

RHANGOS, W. C., and CHICK, E. W. (1964), *Southern Medical Journal*, **57**, 664.

Sporotrichosis. Infection with *Sporotrichum schenkii*, found world wide, is usually limited to the skin and lymph-nodes. The organism is found in plants and is acquired by the prick of a thorn or through minor trauma. An ulcer develops with cord-like thickening of lymphatics, subcutaneous nodules along the path of lymphatics, and lymphadenopathy. Rarely the infection becomes disseminated. Men who work with soil or plants are particularly liable to be affected. Arthritis is monarticular or polyarticular and affects knee, elbow, and small joints of hands or feet usually asymmetrically. Joints are painful, swollen, warm, and tender with effusion and synovial thickening. Untreated arthritis progresses to joint destruction and sinuses may develop. X-ray shows patchy porosis adjacent to the joint; later there is loss of joint space and destruction of joint surfaces. Synovial fluid is inflammatory with raised W.B.C., predominantly neutrophils. Diagnosis is confirmed by culturing the fungus from synovial fluid, biopsy material, or skin lesions.

Treatment: Amphotericin B (*see below*), and excision of granulomatous tissue.

REFERENCES

MIKKELSEN, W. M., and others (1957), *Annals of Internal Medicine*, **47**, 435.

WEBSTER, F. S., and WILLANDER, D. (1957), *Journal of Bone and Joint Surgery*, **39A**, 207.

FUNGUS INFECTIONS (*continued*)

Actinomycosis of bone results from local spread; disease of the mandible follows cervicofacial actinomycosis, and disease of the spine follows abdominal actinomycosis. Arthritis of a proximal interphalangeal or metacarpophalangeal joint may follow a punch, the organism being acquired from the teeth of the opponent. There is a local tender inflamed swelling which breaks down, discharging pus containing 'sulphur granules'. X-ray shows an area of bone destruction adjacent to the joint. The diagnosis is confirmed by microscopy and culture of discharge from the area.

Treatment: Penicillin is effective, but large doses (up to 12 megaunits daily) are sometimes required. Treatment should be continued for about 1 year to prevent relapse. Surgical drainage is required for extensive lesions.

Amphotericin B is very toxic and should be given in a dosage of 50 mg. twice weekly, intravenously in saline over 6 hours, for 1 month.

REFERENCE

WEARNE, W. M. (1960), *Proceedings of the Royal Society of Medicine*, **53**, 884.

GAMEKEEPER'S THUMB

Acute arthritis of the first metacarpophalangeal joint of the thumb caused by injury to the ulnar collateral ligament. This injury is seen in gamekeepers and poachers who kill rabbits with their hands. It may also be the result of a fall, for example, while skiing. There is pain and swelling of the joint with tenderness, particularly on the ulnar side. Lateral instability of the joint may be detectable on clinical examination and can be confirmed by XR. Immobilization in plaster is sufficient treatment for most cases; for the few who fail to respond, surgical repair of the collateral ligament is required.

REFERENCE

British Medical Journal (1974), **1**, 213.

GAUCHER'S DISEASE

A rare condition transmitted as an autosomal recessive character, occurring often, but not always in Jews, characterized by the accumulation of kerasin and other cerebrosides in reticulo-endothelial cells. The characteristic histological feature is the Gaucher cell, a large cell with an eccentric nucleus and pale 'wrinkled' cytoplasm. Arthritis is caused by deposits of Gaucher cells in bone and resultant avascular necrosis. Severity is variable and mild cases may present in old age.

Incidence

M. = F.
Any age, peak 3–20.
About 50 per cent present with bone or joint pain; most develop skeletal problems eventually.

Joints affected

Hip commonest (80 per cent).
Rarely shoulders, ankles, knees, spine, and temporomandibular joint.
70 per cent unilateral; may become bilateral with subsequent episodes.

Symptoms

Pain and stiffness; may begin suddenly or insidiously.

Signs

Painful limitation of movement.
Hip held in flexion and adduction with limb shortening.

Course

Episodes of arthritis recur, often years apart. Untreated, hip involvement progresses to complete destruction of the joint, with secondary osteoarthritis.

Associations

1. Gross splenomegaly; moderate hepatomegaly; hypersplenism.
2. Pigmentation of exposed areas and lower legs.
3. Pingueculae.
4. Pathological fractures, especially of the femur.

XR

Changes may be seen in any bone but are commonest in the femur:
1. Areas of porosis or sclerosis which may or may not be sharply defined.
2. Avascular necrosis.
3. Fractures of long bones; compression fractures of vertebral bodies.
4. Enlargement of the lower end of the femur: expanded porotic medula; thin cortex (Erlenmeyer flask appearance).

Laboratory

Anaemia; sometimes leucopenia and thrombocytopenia.
Biopsy of bone, bone-marrow, or spleen shows Gaucher cells.
Raised acid phosphatase.

Treatment

1. Bed-rest, immobilization in plaster, no weight-bearing and traction for early disease, especially in children, may restore the femoral head to normal. Assess progress with serial X-rays.
2. Splenectomy may be required for hypersplenism or if the spleen is uncomfortably large but has no effect on bone lesions.
3. Radiotherapy may provide pain relief in the difficult case.
4. Surgery in advanced cases with joint destruction.

REFERENCES

ADLER, E., and MAYBAUM, S. (1954), *Annals of the Rheumatic Diseases*, 13, 229.

AMSTUTZ, H. C., and CAREY, E. J. (1966), *Journal of Bone and Joint Surgery*, 48A, 670.

GENU AMORIS

A painful swollen knee caused or aggravated by sexual intercourse in an unusual position. It seems to occur in persons predisposed by some joint disease such as chondromalacia patella and in the enthusiastic, being related to repeated trauma. Though described in the knee, it could occur in other joints in enterprising patients. It is worth remembering sex as well as more conventional traumata such as sport.

REFERENCE

PINALS, R. S. (1976), *Arthritis and Rheumatism*, 19, 637.

GLANDERS

Infection with *Bacillus mallei*, a rare condition particularly of young adult males whose occupation brings them into close contact with horses. There is a chronic septicaemic illness with cutaneous and muscular abscesses, pneumonitis and lung abscess, lymphadenopathy and fever. Arthritis is rare, usually monarticular and affects the large joints, most commonly the knee. Blood-culture is usually negative, but the diagnosis is confirmed by an agglutination test or skin test. The organism may be cultured from abscesses. Treatment: Sulphadiazine.

REFERENCE

ROBINS, G. D. (1906), *Studies from the Royal Victoria Hospital, Montreal*, 2, No. 1.

GONOCOCCAL ARTHRITIS

Arthritis due to gonococcal infection of the joints. The illness may be divided into two stages. In the first or bacteraemic stage there is fever, polyarthritis, and positive blood culture. In the second or septic joint stage, one or two joints are involved and purulent fluid may be aspirated from them. This is to be distinguished from Reiter's disease (*see* p. 110) in which arthritis is often associated with, but not due to, gonococcal infection. Useful points in favour of gonococcal polyarthritis include the female sex, involvement of upper limb as well as lower limb joints, pustular skin lesions, and response to antibiotics.

Incidence
F. 4 : 1.
Any age but particularly young adults, age 15–40.
Often homosexual men, occasionally pregnant women, rarely neonates.
0·2 per cent of cases of gonococcal urethritis develop arthritis.
Arthritis begins 3–17 (usually about 14) days after gonococcal infection.

Joints affected
Polyarticular (75 per cent), usually two to four joints.
Asymmetrical (80 per cent).
Knee commonest (75 per cent).
Often wrist and ankles (40 per cent).
Occasionally elbow, shoulder, hands, feet, and hips.
Rarely vertebrae.

Symptoms
Sudden onset of severe pain and swelling.
Generalized arthralgia often precedes arthritis, associated with fever and rigors.

Signs
Warmth, erythema, tenderness and swelling of joint and periarticular soft tissues.
Effusion usual.
Fever (90 per cent).

Course
Untreated, most patients develop chronic synovitis and eventually deformities.

Effective treatment produces complete resolution within 1–4 weeks.

Associations
1. Tenosynovitis (30 per cent) usually around the wrist.
2. Skin lesions: (70 per cent of cases) crops of lesions which may be maculopapular, haemorrhagic, vesicular, or pustular, particularly on extremities.
3. Other systemic localizations (very rare): endocarditis, meningitis, or conjunctivitis.

XR
Normal in acute stage.
Chronic: may show loss of joint space, erosions, and later joint destruction.

Laboratory
Blood: mild leucocytosis. Slightly raised E.S.R.
Synovial fluid: turbid. Polymorph leucocytosis. Positive culture in 50 per cent.
Organism may also be recovered from blood, genital tract, anus, or pharynx.
Gonococcal-complement fixation test of little value; positive in less than 50 per cent.

Treatment
1. Penicillin (procaine penicillin 1·2 megaunits + benzylpenicillin 1 megaunit daily for 5 days).
2. For sensitivity, resistance, or failure, tetracycline 250 mg. q.d.s. for 7 days.

REFERENCES

HOLMES, K. K., and others (1971), *Annals of Internal Medicine*, 74, 979.

SEIFERT, M. H., and others (1974), *Annals of Rheumatic Diseases*, 33, 140.

GOUT

A disorder of purine metabolism, characterized by hyperuricaemia and the deposition of monosodium urate crystals in joints, resulting in acute attacks of arthritis. In the later stage there is deposition of urate in soft tissues and the kidney, with a chronic arthritis.

Incidence
M. 20 : 1.
Age 30–60 (mean 40). Later (postmenopause) in women.
Upper social classes.
Commoner in Maoris and other Polynesian races.
50 per cent regular alcohol drinkers.
30 per cent have a positive F.H.

Joints affected
Big toe in 75 per cent of attacks.
Occasionally ankle, other toes, knee, or fingers.
Others rare.
One joint in 90 per cent of attacks.

Symptoms
Prodromal irritability. Sudden onset of severe pain, most often at 3–6 a.m. Attacks precipitated by surgery, trauma, dietary or alcoholic excess, starvation, and drugs (salicylates, thiazides, frusemide, and pyrazinamide).

Signs
Red, hot, swollen, exquisitely tender joint.
Local oedema.
Fever common in acute attacks.
Between attacks joints are normal until the chronic or tophaceous stage when urate deposits appear.
20 per cent have tophi, characteristically in the ear-lobe but also around joints.

Course
Untreated acute attacks last for a few days or weeks, and recur at irregular intervals sometimes many years apart.
Later arthritis becomes chronic with tophaceous deposits. In this stage deformities may occur.

Associations
1. Obesity (50 per cent).
2. Hypertension (50 per cent), vascular disease, and renal failure.
3. Renal uric acid stones.

Variants
1. *Secondary gout* accounts for 5 per cent of cases, most due to myeloproliferative disorders particularly polycythaemia rubra vera. Also occurs during treatment of malignant disease. Features are later age of onset (mean 60), less marked male preponderance (only 2 : 1), and absence of family history. Attacks tend to be atypical in site and prolonged. Allopurinol provides useful prophylaxis.
2. *Renal failure* is a very rare cause of gout. Tubular disorders which cause gout are (*a*) lead poisoning (saturnine gout) usually associated with chronic renal failure and proteinuria and often mental impairment; (*b*) hyperparathyroidism; (*c*) hypothyroidism.
3. *Lesch-Nyhan syndrome.* X-borne intermediate inherited deficiency of hypoxanthine-guanine phosphoribosyl transferase (HG PRT-ase). Homozygotes develop spasticity, choreo-athetosis, self-mutilation, and gout in childhood. Heterozygotes develop gout at age 10–30; diagnosis by uric acid excretion (uric acid/creatinine ratio >0.76) confirmed by low erythrocyte HG PRT-ase level.
4. *Glycogen storage disease*, type 1 (von Gierke's disease). Gout occurs after age 14 in those who survive.

XR
Normal in early attacks.
'Punched-out' radiolucent areas around affected joints in the tophaceous stage.

Laboratory
1. Synovial fluid and tophaceous deposits contain needle-shaped crystals which are strongly negatively birefringent.
2. Uric acid usually greater than 6 mg./100 ml. (0·36 mmol./l.) but hyperuricaemia is also found in many other conditions.
3. Raised E.S.R. and leucocytosis in acute attacks.

GOUT (continued)

Treatment

A. *Acute attacks.* Respond rapidly to indomethacin 50–100 mg. stat., then 25–50 mg. t.d.s., phenylbutazone 600–800 mg. on day 1 reducing to 300 mg. daily or colchicine 1 mg. stat., then 0·5 mg. hourly up to 8 mg. or diarrhoea. If no response consider ACTH. Naproxen and fenoprofen are also effective.

B. When completely better, start long-term treatment with allopurinol.

Indications

1. Frequent attacks.
2. Serum uric acid > 9 mg. per 100 ml. (0·54 mmol./l.)
3. Any tophi.
4. Renal stones.

Precautions

1. Start with 100 mg. daily and increase slowly to 300 mg. in a single daily dose. Adjust maintenance dose according to serum uric acid level.
2. Prophylactic colchicine 0·5 mg. b.d. for 3 months.

Uricosuric drugs, e.g., probenecid, may be used as an alternative to allopurinol or in addition in the difficult case.

REFERENCES

EMMERSON, B. T. (1968), *Arthritis and Rheumatism,* **11,** 623.

GRAHAME, R., and SCOTT, J. T. (1970), *Annals of the Rheumatic Diseases,* **29,** 461.

DE SEZE, S., and RYCKEWAERT, A. (1960), *Expansion Scientifique Française.*

YU, T. F., and GUTMAN, A. B. (1959), *Archives of Interamerican Rheumatology,* **2,** 225.

GUINEA-WORM ARTHRITIS (Dracontiasis)

Infection with the nematode, *Dracunculus medinensis,* is acquired by ingestion of water containing infected water fleas (cyclops). Larvae penetrate the intestinal wall and migrate to the subcutaneous tissues. The mature female worm discharges its larvae through the skin, usually of the lower leg or foot, forming first a blister then an ulcer which may become secondarily infected. The condition is found in parts of Africa, South America, India, Burma, Persia, and Turkey. Arthritis is due to the presence of a worm and the discharge of its larvae within the joint.

Incidence

M. = F.
Any age, peak in young adults.

Joints affected

Knee usually.
Monarticular.

Symptoms

Sudden onset of pain and swelling.
Patient may have 'felt something moving' in the subcutaneous tissues before the development of arthritis.

Signs

Swollen, warm, tender joint with marked limitation of movement and effusion.
Later synovial thickening.
Fever usual.

Course

Untreated, the condition is chronic and progresses slowly to a chronic synovitis and eventually joint destruction or ankylosis.

Associations

Generalized pruritus, urticaria, nausea and vomiting, diarrhoea, asthma, malaise, weakness, and fever, preceding the arthritis by a few days.

XR

Normal.
Calcified worms are occasionally seen in the skin.

Laboratory

W.B.C.: eosinophilia.
Synovial fluid: turbid; mixed cellular infiltrate; microscopy shows guinea-worm larvae.

Treatment

1. Exploration of the joint and removal of worms and larvae.
2. Niridazole (25 mg. per kg. per day in two doses for 7 days) kills all worms; worms in skin may then be extracted.
3. Antibiotics for secondary infection.

REFERENCE

REDDY, C. R. R. M., and SIVARAMAPPA, M. (1968), *British Medical Journal,* **1,** 155.

HAEMANGIOMA

Haemangioma of the synovial membrane is a rare benign tumour of joints affecting particularly children and young adults. The knee is the commonest site (95 per cent). Symptoms and signs vary according to whether the condition is diffuse or localized.

Diffuse: the joint is swollen and there may be episodes of pain associated with haemarthrosis. There may also be enlargement of the limb. On examination the swelling is typically 'doughy', compressible and may be reduced by elevation of the limb. The joint is sometimes warm and tender and there is occasionally a haemangioma of the overlying skin.

Localized: there are episodes of pain, locking and 'giving way' suggestive of a mechanical derangement. Swelling is localized to part of the joint and may appear and disappear.

The diagnosis is usually suggested by the finding of blood-stained synovial fluid and confirmed by arthroscopy.

Treatment: Excision is successful for the localized variety. With the diffuse variety, recurrence is common and it should therefore be treated conservatively.

REFERENCE

HALBORG, A., and others (1968), *Acta Orthopaedica Scandinavica*, **39**, 1223.

HAEMARTHROSIS

Haemorrhage into a joint may arise from any of the following causes:

1. Trauma including surgery.
2. Villonodular synovitis (p. 97).
3. Scurvy (p. 122).
4. Haemangioma (*see above*).
5. Malignant tumours in or around joints. Leukaemia.
6. Anticoagulant therapy—usually one knee or ankle in a patient on an oral anticoagulant.
7. Haemophilia and Christmas disease (p. 42).
8. Idiopathic joint apoplexy.
9. Crystal deposition disease—occasionally a haemorrhagic effusion is found in patients with acute gout or pseudogout.

REFERENCE

COHEN, G. L., and others (1969), *Arthritis and Rheumatism*, **12**, 287.

HAEMOCHROMATOSIS

Hereditary disorder of iron metabolism transmitted as an autosomal intermediate and characterized by iron deposition in the liver, endocrine glands, heart, and synovial membranes. Two types of arthropathy occur: (1) A chronic arthropathy particularly affecting the hands. (2) Pyrophosphate arthropathy (*see* p. 108).

Incidence

M. 10 : 1.
Onset age 20+, peak 40–60.
50 per cent develop arthropathy; commoner in those aged 50+. Joint symptoms usually begin at the same time or up to 20 years after other manifestations but in 15 per cent arthropathy precedes. F.H. rare but relatives have *forme fruste*.

Joints affected

Small joints of hands: second and third M.C.P. joints usually involved, first, fourth, and fifth often.
20 per cent have more widespread arthropathy affecting hips and other large joints.

Symptoms

Mild pain and limitation of movement.

Signs

Bony swelling.
Limitation of movement.

Course

Chronic progressive arthropathy but deformity and disability are rare.
No response to venesection.
30 per cent have acute attacks of pyrophosphate arthropathy during course of disease.

HAEMOCHROMATOSIS (*continued*)

Associations
1. Pigmentation.
2. Loss of body hair, diminished sexual activity.
3. Hepatomegaly (often painful or tender). Liver carcinoma in 15 per cent.
4. Diabetes mellitus (80 per cent).
5. High alcohol intake.
6. Heart failure or arrhythmia (30 per cent).

XR
1. Joint narrowing, subarticular cysts and sclerosis of joint margins, best seen in M.C.P. joints.
2. Chondrocalcinosis.

Laboratory
Raised serum iron.
Increased saturation of total iron binding capacity (>60 per cent).
Liver biopsy shows iron deposition.
Glucose-tolerance test.

Treatment
1. Analgesics.
2. Venesection (1 or 2 pints weekly for 2 years) improves pigmentation, diabetes, liver function, and heart failure but not arthropathy or sexual function.
3. Insulin. Testosterone.

REFERENCES
DYMOCK, I. W., and others (1970), *Annals of Rheumatic Diseases*, **29**, 469.

SHERLOCK, S. (1968), *Diseases of the Liver and Biliary System*, 4th ed. Oxford: Blackwell.

HAEMOPHILIA

Rare disorder of the blood-clotting mechanism caused by deficiency of Factor VIII, inherited as an X-linked recessive character. Attacks of arthritis are due to haemorrhage into joints and also occur in *Christmas disease* and other rarer deficiencies. Acute haemarthrosis may be associated with other haemorrhagic conditions, e.g., overdosage with anticoagulant drugs and after trauma. Recurrent haemarthroses lead to a degenerative arthropathy which is characteristic of haemophilia.

Incidence
Almost all males.
Onset usually in the first few years of life; rarely in later childhood or adolescence.
90 per cent have attacks of arthritis; common presenting feature.
F.H. of haemophilia in 70 per cent.

Joints affected
Knee commonest (70 per cent).
Elbow or ankle in 20 per cent.
Occasionally shoulder, hip, or wrist.
Monarticular in 70 per cent.
Asymmetrical.

Symptoms
Sudden onset of very severe pain, sometimes after mild trauma which may be minimal.
Occasionally pain is mild or absent and it is important to treat such attacks in the same way.

Signs
Joint is red, warm, swollen, and very tender; the limb is held immobile, often in flexion with marked muscle spasm.
After repeated attacks there is bony swelling, permanent limitation of movement, crepitus, often deformities (flexion contractures of knees and elbows commonest), and marked muscle wasting.

Course
Recurrent acute attacks especially in childhood.
Complete recovery at first but later deformities and degenerative changes develop.

Associations
Other internal haemorrhages.

XR
Normal with early attacks.
Later small irregular superficial erosions and cysts appear.
Later still loss of joint space, sclerosis, flattening of joint surfaces, and sometimes bizarre disorganization of the joint.
Epiphyseal changes may be seen in children.

Laboratory
Normal blood-count, platelets, and prothrombin time.
Prolonged partial thromboplastin time; confirm by Factor VIII assay.
Blood-stained synovial fluid.

HAEMOPHILIA (*continued*)

Treatment

1. Complete immobilization in acute stage. Plaster cast usually required in children.
2. Factor VIII. Cryoprecipitate or fresh plasma. Treatment should be started as soon as possible.
3. Analgesics. Narcotics often required. Local ice packs may help.
4. Aspiration unnecessary and best avoided in most cases; may speed recovery in cases with large tense effusions.
5. Gentle physiotherapy to restore range of movement after acute stage.
6. Later correction of deformities and rehabilitation.

Prophylaxis: avoid even trivial trauma.

Variants

Haemorrhage into muscles around joints causes a similar picture; pain is even more severe and contractures may result.

REFERENCES

FRANCE, W. G., and WOLF, P. (1965), *Journal of Bone and Joint Surgery*, **47B**, 247.

JORDAN, H. H. (1958), *Haemophilic Arthropathies*. Thomas: Springfield, Ill.

HANDIGODU SYNDROME

A rare disorder affecting only people of the Malnad area of the state of Karnataka in South India. It is named after the village in which an 'epidemic' of about 30 cases appeared in 1975. Symptoms usually begin between ages 4 and 20 (up to 40) with pain in the hips or knees. Both hips and both knees are eventually involved with spine, ankles, shoulders, elbows or wrists affected later in about one-third of cases. The hips are usually most severely affected with painful limitation of movement. Joints are only occasionally swollen. XR of hip-joints show premature closure of epiphysis, loss of joint space, irregular joint surfaces, sclerosis, cysts and osteophytes, sometimes with flattening of the femoral head. Similar changes are seen in the knees, where they are less severe, and less commonly in other affected joints. E.S.R. is not raised. Effusions are not found and synovial fluid is normal. The disease progresses in severe cases to cause great disability with restriction of movement and fixed flexion deformity requiring surgery.

REFERENCE

MANI, K. S., and SRINIVASA MURTHY, H. K. National Institute of Mental Health and Neuro Sciences, Bangalore. Personal communication.

HEMIPLEGIA

A transient arthritis affecting hemiplegic limbs. In contrast, the joints of paralysed limbs are either less severely affected or spared by rheumatoid arthritis and osteoarthritis.

Incidence

Onset 1 to 5 weeks after stroke.
Age over 60.
M. = F.

Joints affected

Knee, ankle, wrist, shoulder, or elbow. From 1 to 3 joints are affected, usually only in the paralysed limbs.

Symptoms

Sudden onset of pain and swelling.

Signs

Effusion, warmth, and tenderness.

Course

Arthritis resolves completely in 2 to 6 weeks. No residua.

Associations

Hemiplegia or hemiparesis sometimes complicated by respiratory or urinary tract infection.

XR

No specific changes but degenerative changes are common in this age-group.

Laboratory

Raised E.S.R.; slight leucocytosis. Latex test negative.

Synovial fluid: Inflammatory and sometimes turbid. W.B.C. up to 20,000 × 10⁹/dl., predominantly neutrophils.
Sterile on culture.

Treatment
Anti-inflammatory drugs.
Aspiration of fluid and injection of steroid may speed recovery.

REFERENCE

HERMANN, E. (1972), *Scandinavian Journal of Rheumatology*, 1, 87.

HENOCH-SCHÖNLEIN PURPURA (Anaphylactoid Purpura)

A condition characterized by an exanthem with either gastro-intestinal manifestations or arthritis or both. The association of arthritis and purpura was first described by Schönlein. The condition may follow upper respiratory-tract infection, often streptococcal. Biopsy of skin lesions shows a characteristic perivascular acute inflammatory reaction often with eosinophilic infiltration.

Incidence
M. 3 : 1.
Peak age 3–15; rare in adults.
Arthritis in 75 per cent, synchronous with skin lesions.

Joints affected
Knees and ankles commonest.
Often elbows, wrists, and hips.
Occasionally small joints of hands or feet.
Bilateral and symmetrical; only rarely migratory.

Symptoms
Presents with rash, colic or joint pains, commonly following within 2 weeks after an upper respiratory-tract infection.
Pain often severe; joints stiff and swollen.

Signs
Often none.
Sometimes periarticular soft-tissue swelling, tenderness and effusion.
Slight fever common.

Course
Arthritis usually lasts only a few days but up to 1 week.
Other manifestations last up to 6 weeks and resolve completely except with renal manifestations when the illness may be prolonged.

Associations
1. The rash is at first urticarial and itching, then maculopapular with lesions up to 2 cm. in diameter changing from pink to deep purple, becoming brown and fading over about 2 weeks but recurring in 'crops'.
Typically found on the buttocks and extensor surfaces.
Occasionally there are petechiae, ecchymoses, or patches of oedema, usually around the eyes.
2. Gastro-intestinal manifestations in 60 per cent: colic, vomiting, gastro-intestinal bleeding.
Intussusception or perforation may result.
3. Gross or microscopic haematuria in 40 per cent; most cases recover but rarely progress to renal failure or chronic nephritis. Residual albuminuria in 10 per cent which often disappears over the years.

XR
Normal.

Laboratory
E.S.R. raised.
Platelets and clotting tests normal.
Throat swab: haemolytic streptococcus (25 per cent): ASO titre raised (35 per cent).
Biopsy of skin lesion shows characteristic changes.
Synovial fluid: viscous with raised W.B.C., mainly polymorphs.

Treatment
Salicylates or other non-steroidal anti-inflammatory drugs. Not steroids.

REFERENCE

BYWATERS, E. G. L., and others (1957), *Quarterly Journal of Medicine*, 26, 161.

CHRONIC ACTIVE HEPATITIS (Lupoid Hepatitis; Juvenile Cirrhosis)

A type of chronic progressive liver disease common in young females. The condition overlaps with S.L.E. (*see* p. 132) in the finding of L.E. cells and other manifestations in some cases; but the disease remains predominantly a liver disease throughout its course.

Incidence
F. 5 : 1.
Any age; peak 10–30.
30 per cent have joint pains, usually early in the course of the disease and rarely preceding other manifestations by a few months.
Onset usually coincides with exacerbation of liver disease.

Joints affected
Polyarticular.
P.I.P. and M.C.P. joints, wrists, knees, ankles, and elbows commonest.
Bilateral and symmetrical.

Symptoms
Pain and stiffness.
Morning stiffness.

Signs
Sometimes none; sometimes soft-tissue swelling.
Joints are only rarely red, hot, or tender.
Fever often.

Course
Usually transient but, rarely, chronic and progressive, resembling rheumatoid arthritis.
Responds to steroids.
Hypertension and liver failure develop often within a few years; death common within 10 years.

Associations
1. Persistent jaundice. Onset often mistaken for infectious hepatitis.
2. Splenomegaly in 90 per cent, hepatomegaly variable.
3. Cutaneous striae, spider naevi, or acne in 60 per cent.
4. Amenorrhoea in females (70 per cent). Gynaecomastia in males.
5. Sjögren's syndrome (30 per cent).
6. Occasionally other manifestations of S.L.E. (*see* p. 132), e.g., nephritis or rashes.

XR
Usually normal. Rarely erosions and narrowing of joint space.

Laboratory
Raised serum bilirubin (2–10 mg. per cent = 35–170 µmol./l.) mixed conjugated and unconjugated.
Persistently raised transaminases.
Smooth-muscle antibody usually present; mitochondrial antibody in 30 per cent.
Latex test and A.N.F. positive in 80 per cent.
L.E. cells in 50 per cent.
Hypergammaglobulinaemia.
Synovial fluid: non-inflammatory.

Treatment
1. Prednisolone 30 mg. daily, reducing to a maintenance dose of about 15 mg. daily.
2. Consider immunosuppressive drugs for persistent activity or steroid side-effects.

REFERENCE

WHELTON, M. J. (1970), *British Journal of Hospital Medicine*, 3, 243.

HEREDITARY ANGIO-OEDEMA

A rare condition inherited as an autosomal dominant, characterized by recurrent episodes of subcutaneous swelling, abdominal pain, and diarrhoea. The swellings cause discomfort and sometimes pain; they may occur over joints, and the condition has been mistaken for palindromic rheumatism. The diagnosis is confirmed by finding absence of the normal inhibitor of the complement fraction C1 in plasma. Treatment of the acute attack: Fresh plasma. ε-amino caproic acid prevents attacks.

REFERENCE

WEBB, F. W. S. (1970), *Proceedings of the Royal Society of Medicine*, 63, 281.

HEREDITARY PROGRESSIVE ARTHRO-OPHTHALMOPATHY

A rare condition, inherited as an autosomal dominant, characterized by myopia and a degenerative arthropathy.

Incidence
M. = F.
Onset in childhood.
Most cases have arthropathy.

Joints affected
Knees commonest; also ankles, wrists, elbows, shoulders, hips, and spine.
Occasionally M.C.P. joints.
Onset in one joint spreading to involve many; eventually bilateral and symmetrical.

Symptoms
Stiffness and pain after exertion. Later, persistent pain and 'locking'.

Signs
Bony swelling characteristic.
Joints occasionally red and warm in exacerbations.
Hypermobility common.
Late: limitation of motion and crepitus.
Thoracic kyphosis common.

Course
Chronic progressive course eventually causing severe painful limitation of movement.

Associations
1. High myopia leading to total retinal detachment and blindness in the first decade of life; later the eyes develop cataract and iritis.
2. Congenital skeletal deformities are rarely present.

XR
1. Irregularity of joint surfaces with wide joint space.
2. Abnormal shapes of bones, e.g., flattening of articular surfaces.
3. Loose bodies.
4. Late stage resembles severe osteoarthritis with narrowing of joint space and sclerosis.
5. Spine: anterior wedging and flattening of vertebrae.

Laboratory
E.S.R. may be raised.
Synovial biopsy shows no evidence of inflammation.

Treatment
Analgesics.

REFERENCES

STICKLER, G. B., and PUGH, D. G. (1967) *Proceedings of Staff Meetings of the Mayo Clinic*, **42**, 495.

STICKLER, G. B., and others (1965), *Proceedings of Staff Meetings of the Mayo Clinic*, **40**, 433.

HEREDITARY VASCULAR AND ARTICULAR CALCIFICATION

A rare condition inherited as an autosomal recessive character, in which recurrent attacks of joint pain and swelling are accompanied by radiological calcification of joints and blood-vessels. Heterozygotes may have vascular calcification but not arthritis.

Incidence

M.=F.
Onset in young adults.

Joints affected

One or several.
Small joints of hands commonest.
Sometimes feet, ankles, knees, wrists, elbows, manubriosternal, and sternoclavicular joints.

Symptoms

Attacks of joint pain and swelling.

Signs

Joints are red, warm, and swollen in the acute stage.
This settles, leaving only bony swelling.
Limitation of movement and crepitus develop over the years.

Course

Attacks last for a few weeks and recur at irregular intervals months or years apart.
Disability is mild.

Associations

Palpable nodular arteries; diminished or absent pulses.

XR

1. Calcification of blood-vessels.
2. Calcium deposition in joint capsule; new bone formation around joints, especially small joints of hands.
3. Erosions.
4. Ligamentous calcification in the spine resembling ankylosing spondylitis. Sacro-iliac joints may be normal or may show irregularity, sclerosis, or fusion.

Laboratory

Calcium, phosphates, alkaline phosphatase, and E.S.R. normal.

Treatment

Analgesics when required.

REFERENCE

SHARP, J. (1954), *Annals of the Rheumatic Diseases*, **13, 15.**

HERPES ZOSTER

Infection of the posterior root ganglion with the varicella virus, causing pain in the segmental distribution of the affected root followed by a vesicular rash in the same distribution. Two types of arthritis occur, both rare:

1. Arthritis of the small joints of the hand in the distribution of affected nerves.
2. Shoulder–hand syndrome (*see* p. 125).

Incidence

M. = F.
Any age, but particularly over 50.
Arthritis is a rare complication and occurs particularly in cases with paralysis; synchronous with skin lesions.

Joints affected

Small joints of hands or wrist.
Unilateral—confined to the side of the skin lesions.

Symptoms

Severe pain and swelling.

Signs

Swelling, tenderness, painful restriction of movement, and oedema of peri-articular soft-tissues.

Course

Lasts for months and is often followed by contractures and limitation of movement of affected joints.

Associations

1. Vesicular rash confined to one or more dermatomes, lasting for about 1 week before scabs are formed which heal with scarring.
2. Rash is often preceded and sometimes followed by intense burning pain in the same distribution.
3. Rare complications include motor paralysis resembling poliomyelitis, meningo-encephalitis, and tenosynovitis.

XR

Normal or peri-articular porosis.

Laboratory

No characteristic findings.

Treatment

1. Symptomatic: aspirin.
2. Prevention of deformities.

REFERENCE

QUIN, C. E. (1973), *Rheumatology and Rehabilitation*, **12**, 74.

HISTOPLASMOSIS

Dust-borne infection with the fungus *Histoplasma capsulatum*, found particularly in the U.S.A. Infection is usually manifest as a pulmonary illness resembling tuberculosis. It rarely becomes disseminated causing hepatosplenomegaly and metastatic infection elsewhere. Arthritis is of two types:
1. Associated with the initial pulmonary infection and erythema nodosum or erythema multiforme. This may be sporadic or epidemic.[1]

Incidence

F. 6 : 1.
Any age, peak 35–65.

Joints affected

Feet, ankles, knees, spine, and hands commonest.
Often migratory.

Symptoms

Pain, often severe, worst in the early morning, improving during the day.

Signs

Joints are swollen but only occasionally warm or red.

Course

Arthritis lasts up to 2 months, and resolves completely without residua.

Associations

1. Erythema nodosum or erythema multiforme or both.
2. Conjunctivitis (50 per cent). Iritis.

XR

Normal.
CXR may show patchy infiltration.

Laboratory

Raised E.S.R.
Diagnosis confirmed by positive complement-fixation test, agglutination test, or histoplasmin skin-test.

Treatment

Anti-inflammatory drugs.

2. Bone and joint involvement in disseminated infection is very rare. Monarticular arthritis of the wrist and knee has been reported. Treatment: Amphotericin B. Excision of infected material may be required.[2]

REFERENCES

[1] SELLORS, T. F., and others (1965), *Annals of Internal Medicine*, **62**, 1244.

[2] OMER, G. E., and others (1963), *Journal of Bone and Joint Surgery*, **45A**, 1699.

HOFFA'S DISEASE (Lipoarthritis Traumatica Genu)

Pain in the knee-joint arising from the infrapatellar pad of fat. The condition occurs particularly in ballet dancers and acrobats, and is due to incarceration of the fringes of the fat pad in the joint. Pain follows a traumatic episode, may continue for months, and is completely relieved by excision of the fat pad. There is tenderness below the patella, but the knee-joint is otherwise normal.

REFERENCE

NILSONNE, H. (1931), *Acta Orthopaedica Scandinavica*, **2**, 318.

HYPERLIPOPROTEINAEMIA (Type 2)

A rare, genetically determined disorder of cholesterol metabolism, transmitted as an autosomal intermediate, characterized in homozygotes by marked elevation of plasma cholesterol, xanthomatosis, and atherosclerosis occurring at an early age.

Incidence
M. = F.
Onset age 5–10.
50 per cent of homozygotes develop arthritis.
Not heterozygotes.

Joints affected
Large joints, knees commonest: also ankles, hips, elbows, and wrists.
Often migratory, each joint being affected for a day or two.

Symptoms
Acute onset of pain and swelling.

Signs
None in mild attacks.
Severely affected joints are warm, tender, and swollen with marked limitation of movement.
Fever common.

Course
Attacks of arthritis last up to 1 week and recur at irregular intervals, often years apart.

Associations
1. Tuberous, tendinous, and periosteal xanthomata; xanthelasmata; corneal arcus.
2. Premature atherosclerosis.
3. Cardiac murmurs, usually aortic systolic. Note resemblance to rheumatic fever (age, migratory polyarthritis, murmurs), but no evidence of preceding streptococcal infection.

XR
Usually normal.
Erosions of phalanges not usually involving the joint surface have been described.

Laboratory
Raised plasma cholesterol.
E.S.R. raised in attacks.

Treatment
Symptomatic; salicylates.
Low cholesterol and saturated, high polyunsaturated fat diet; cholestyramine.

REFERENCES

FREDRICKSON, D. S., and others (1967), *New England Journal of Medicine*, **276**, 34.
MARCH, H. C., and others (1957), *American Journal of Roentgenology*, **77**, 109.
KHACHADURIAN, A. K. (1968), *Arthritis and Rheumatism*, **11**, 385.

HYPERLIPOPROTEINAEMIA (Type 4)

A metabolic disorder characterized by increased levels of endogenous triglycerides (preβ-lipoproteins). The condition may be inherited as an autosomal dominant and is aggravated by alcohol and obesity. It is occasionally secondary to hypothyroidism, nephrotic syndromes, oestrogen, oral contraceptives and some rarer diseases. It may be associated with joint symptoms leading to an erroneous diagnosis of palindromic rheumatism, rheumatoid arthritis or psychogenic rheumatism.

Incidence
M. = F.
Age 40–60.
Usually obese.

Joints affected
Pain is usually polyarticular, bilateral and symmetrical. Small and large joints—M.C.P., P.I.P. and D.I.P. joints common.

Symptoms
Pain. Sometimes morning stiffness may be aggravated or precipitated by cold, damp or exertion.

Signs
Often none. One to four joints may be tender and slightly swollen during attacks—usually asymmetrical distribution. Effusion unusual.

Course
Joint disease is neither episodic or chronic with periodic exacerbations. Episodes last for days or weeks. Arthritis may respond to reduction of serum lipid levels. No progressive or permanent joint changes.

Associations
1. Obesity
2. Insulin resistance and glucose intolerance.
3. Vascular disease.
4. Occasionally xanthomata and rarely pancreatitis.

Laboratory
Increased triglycerides.
Increased very low density lipoproteins (pre β-lipoproteins).
No chylomicrons.
Cholesterol normal or slightly raised.
E.S.R. usually normal.
Latex test positive in 50 per cent.
Synovial fluid: 'non-inflammatory'—viscous. W.B.C. up to $10,000 \times 10^9$/dl., mainly mononuclear.
Synovial biopsy: non-specific changes.

XR
Usually normal.
Sometimes porosis or subarticular cysts.

Treatment
1. Diet. Restoration of body weight to ideal. Reduction of carbohydrate and alcohol. Follow triglyceride level.
2. If unsuccessful, low fat diet and clofibrate.
3. Symptomatic therapy for arthritis: rest; analgesic and anti-inflammatory drugs.

REFERENCES

BUCKINGHAM, R. R. and others (1975), *Archives of Internal Medicine*, **135**, 286.

GOLDMAN, J. A. and others (1972), *Lancet*, **2**, 449.

HYPERMOBILITY SYNDROME

Arthropathy associated with joint laxity. Hypermobility is a common finding in children, especially at age 2–3, but seldom persists into adult life; it is a feature of some congenital conditions (*see* p. 53) and may also be acquired in rheumatoid arthritis and other chronic inflammatory arthropathies, neuropathic joints, acromegaly, rheumatic fever, and neurological diseases associated with hypotonicity. The hypermobility syndrome (without other abnormalities) is inherited as an autosomal dominant.

Incidence

M. = F.
Onset in children or young adults with traumatic synovitis or unexplained effusion; or at age 30–50 with premature osteoarthritis.

Joints affected

Knee commonest (70 per cent).
Often hands (thumb base and small joints) or wrists.
Occasionally ankles, cervical or lumbar spine, and feet. Others rare.
One or many joints.

Symptoms

Joint and muscle pains.
Sometimes related to trauma.

Signs

Hypermobility (hyperextension and dorsiflexion of fingers; hyperextension of knees and elbows; flexion of trunk so that hands rest flat on the floor).
Joint effusions; later bony swelling and crepitus.

Course

Osteoarthritic changes progress to moderate disability at older ages.

Associations

Dislocation of shoulder or patella.
Congenital dislocation of hip.

XR

Early: normal.
Later: degenerative changes (loss of joint space, sclerosis, osteophytes, subarticular cysts).

Laboratory

Normal E.S.R.
Synovial fluid: non-inflammatory.

Treatment

1. Analgesics as required.
2. Avoid trauma.

REFERENCES

GRAHAME, R. (1971), *Proceedings of the Royal Society of Medicine*, **64**, 692.

KIRK, J. A., and others (1967), *Annals of the Rheumatic Diseases*, **26**, 419.

CONDITIONS ASSOCIATED WITH HYPERMOBILITY

Marfan's Syndrome[1]

Autosomal dominant inheritance of tall, slender build, long fingers and toes (arachnodactyly), high arched palate, and often other skeletal deformities such as pigeon chest, flat feet, and kyphoscoliosis. 50 per cent have eye defects, most commonly ectopia lentis. 20 per cent have cardiovascular defects: septal defects, conduction defects, and aneurysms. Later manifestations are aortic incompetence and dissecting aneurysm particularly in males. 30 per cent have backache; 20 per cent have arthritis.

Ehlers-Danlos Syndrome[2]

Autosomal dominant inheritance of velvety, fragile, hyperextensible skin (poor healing—tissue-paper scars), easy bruising, and sometimes other congenital abnormalities. Several types are described including a rare ecchymotic type with a tendency to extensive bruising after minor trauma associated with early death from arterial rupture, aortic dissection, or intestinal perforation. Another rare type is transmitted as an X-linked recessive.

Osteogenesis Imperfecta[3]

Autosomal dominant inheritance of bone fragility resulting in recurrent fractures and severe deformities. Severe cases die in utero; mild cases present with fractures and osteoporosis in adult life. Associated abnormalities include a large head, small hands and feet, short limbs, blue sclerae, deafness, and easy bruising. Survival to adult life is unusual.

Bonnevie-Ullrich-Turner Syndrome[3]

A variant of Turner's syndrome: The XO chromosome constitution in females, associated with lymphoedema in infancy, dwarfism, webbing of the neck, amenorrhoea, cardiac, and other congenital abnormalities.

Homocystinuria[4]

Autosomal recessive inheritance of cystathione synthetase deficiency. It resembles Marfan's syndrome with arachnodactyly, slender build, and ectopia lentis but there are also osteoporosis and fractures, arterial or venous thromboses, and often mental retardation.

Marfanoid Hypermobility Syndrome[5]

Arachnodactyly and skeletal features of Marfan's syndrome with skin hyperextensibility without ocular or cardiovascular abnormalities.

Achard Syndrome[6]

Arachnodactyly associated with mandibulofacial dysostosis (broad skull and micrognathism).

Hyperlysinaemia[7]

Very rare syndrome, inherited as an autosomal recessive characterized by mental retardation, arrested physical and sexual development in childhood, epilepsy, and facial abnormalities accompanied by hyperlysinaemia and hyperlysinuria.

Larsen's Syndrome[8]

Autosomal recessive inheritance of characteristic facies (prominent forehead, depressed nasal bridge, and wide-spaced eyes) with joint laxity leading to recurrent dislocations of hips, elbows, knees, and ankles.

Cartilage Hair Hypoplasia[9]

Autosomal recessive inheritance of dwarfism, short stubby hands and feet, short finger-nails, and fine, sparse, fair hair accompanied by metaphysial dysplasia.

Down's Syndrome (mongolism).

Trisomy 21 with dwarfism, mental retardation, characteristic facies, and other limb and heart abnormalities.

REFERENCES

[1] SINCLAIR, R. J. G., and others (1960), *Quarterly Journal of Medicine*, **29**, 19.

[2] BEIGHTON, P., and others (1969), *Annals of the Rheumatic Diseases*, **28**, 228.

[3] McKUSICK, V. A. (1966), *Hereditable Disorders of Connective Tissue*. St. Louis: Mosby.

[4] SCHIMKE, R. N., and others (1965), *Journal of the American Medical Association*, **193**, 711.

[5] WALKER, B. A., and others (1969), *Annals of Internal Medicine*, **71**, 349.

[6] PARISH, J. G. (1960), *Proceedings of the Royal Society of Medicine*, **53**, 515.

[7] GHADIMI, H., and others (1965), *New England Journal of Medicine*, **273**, 723.

[8] STEEL, H. H., and KOHL, E. J. (1972), *Journal of Bone and Joint Surgery*, **54A**, 75.

[9] BEALS, R. K. (1968), *Journal of Bone and Joint Surgery*, **50A**, 1245.

HYPERPARATHYROIDISM

Excessive production of parathormone usually by an autonomous parathyroid adenoma (very rarely hyperplasia or carcinoma). Three types of arthritis occur:
1. *Osteogenic synovitis*, described below, due to softening and collapse of subchondral bone. Arthritis may occur for the same reason in *osteomalacia*.[1]
2. *Pyrophosphate arthropathy* (*see* p. 108) due to hypercalcaemia.[2]
3. *Gout* (*see* p. 39) which results from diminished tubular uric acid secretion.[3]

Incidence
F. 5 : 1.
Onset age 30–70.
Arthritis is a rare presenting feature; may follow parathyroidectomy.

Joints affected
Polyarticular.
Knees commonly involved.
Occasionally spine, hands, feet, wrists, elbows, and ankles.
Often symmetrical resembling rheumatoid arthritis.

Symptoms
Sudden or gradual onset of pain, often severe, worse on weight-bearing. Joints stiff and swollen. Morning stiffness may occur.

Signs
Joints may be red and hot at onset.
Effusion common. Marked tenderness. Crepitus.

Course
Chronic. Untreated, arthritis progresses, sometimes rapidly, to secondary osteo-arthritis which is often disabling.

Associations
1. Anorexia, vomiting, and constipation.
2. Polyuria, polydipsia, and renal colic.
3. Weakness and tiredness.
4. Band keratopathy.
5. Mental changes.

XR
1. Erosions indistinguishable from those of rheumatoid arthritis.
2. Generalized porosis; vertebral collapse; fractures.
3. Subperiosteal resorption along the phalanges, giving a 'saw-tooth' appearance.
4. Lytic lesions.
5. Calcification of cartilage and soft tissues.
6. Bone destruction in later stages of arthropathy, e.g., head of femur.

Laboratory
Raised serum calcium, low phosphates.
Alkaline phosphatase may be raised.
Repeat serum calcium X3 if suspicious.
Raised urea in later stages.
Hyperuricaemia in 50 per cent.
Normal E.S.R. Negative latex test.

Treatment
Exploration of neck and removal of adenoma.
10 per cent have multiple adenomata.
Rarely intrathoracic.

REFERENCES

[1] ZVAIFLER, N. J., and others (1962), *Arthritis and Rheumatism*, **5**, 237.
[2] BYWATERS, E. G. L., and others (1963), *Annals of the Rheumatic Diseases*, **22**, 171.
[3] KISS, Z. S., and others (1967), *Archives of Internal Medicine*, **119**, 279.

HYPOPHOSPHATAEMIC SPONDYLOPATHY

Familial hypophosphataemia is a rare variant of renal or vitamin D-resistant rickets, inherited as an X-borne dominant character. Defective tubular reabsorption of phosphates leads to rickets in childhood, which heals spontaneously at about the age of puberty. In later life, affected individuals may develop spinal stiffness with ligamentous calcification, easily mistaken for ankylosing spondylitis.

Incidence
F. 3 : 1.
Often more severe in men.
Onset after age 20.

Joints affected
Spine, hips, and elbows commonly.
Often also shoulders, knees, wrists, ankles, hands, and feet.

Symptoms
Gradual onset of stiffness and increasing limitation of movement.
Slight morning stiffness.
Pain mild or absent.

Signs
Limitation of movement of spine and affected joints.
No swelling or local tenderness.

Course
Slowly progressive limitation of movement over the years.

Associations
1. Past history of rickets with dwarfism and residual deformities such as bow legs.
2. Fractures and pseudofractures.
3. Severe dental caries.
4. Rarely spinal cord or root compression.

XR
Ligamentous calcification.
New bone formation around the pelvis.
Obliteration of sacro-iliac joints.

Laboratory
Serum phosphates low.
Serum calcium low or normal.
Raised alkaline phosphatase.

Treatment
Symptomatic.

REFERENCES

HART, F. D. (1968), *Lancet*, **1**, 740.

KELLGREN, J. H., and others (1967), *Abstracts of the VIth European Rheumatology Congress*, p. 559.

HYPOTHYROIDISM

Deficiency of thyroid hormone may cause a variety of rheumatic manifestations: (1) Pains and stiffness in proximal muscles. (2) Polyarthritis. (3) Mono-arthritis associated with osteolytic lesions usually in children. (4) Carpal tunnel syndrome. (5) Secondary gout (*see* p. 39). (6) Pains in the neck, shoulders, and upper chest in about 10 per cent of cases of Hashimoto's thyroiditis.

Incidence
F. 3 : 1.
Peak age 40–60.
Arthralgia and myalgia are common; arthritis is rare; carpal tunnel syndrome occurs in 50 per cent.
Arthritis is usually synchronous with other manifestations of hypothyroidism.

Joints affected
Arthralgia and myalgia affect the shoulder and pelvic girdles.
Arthritis usually affects the knees, often wrists, M.T.P., or M.C.P. joints, and occasionally ankles or elbows.
Bilateral and symmetrical except with osteolytic lesions which particularly affect the hip or knee.

Symptoms
Insidious onset of joint pain and stiffness; often severe morning stiffness; aggravated by cold or phenylbutazone therapy.
Acroparaesthesiae due to carpal tunnel syndrome, especially at night.
Muscle cramps common.

Signs
Often none. Affected joints may be swollen with synovial thickening and effusion.

Course
Rheumatic manifestations respond to treatment with thyroxine. No residua.

Associations
1. Tiredness, weakness, weight-gain, constipation, menorrhagia.
2. Goitre.
3. Hoarse voice.
4. Skin changes (dry, coarse, puffy, cold, pale, sometimes yellow); dry, sparse hair.
5. Slow relaxation phase of tendon reflexes; other neuromuscular manifestations include proximal muscle wasting, myotonia, deafness, dementia, and psychosis.
6. Bradycardia; sometimes heart failure, or angina.

XR
Porosis common. Osteolytic lesions rare.

Laboratory
Anaemia; E.S.R. slightly raised.
Confirm diagnosis by raised cholesterol, low P.B.I. or thyroxine level, and abnormal E.C.G.
Look for thyroid antibodies.
Hyperuricaemia common.
Synovial fluid: non-inflammatory.

Treatment
Thyroxine; start with 0·05 mg. daily and increase slowly to maintenance dose of 0·3 mg. daily. Increase very slowly in the elderly and with heart disease.
Avoid phenylbutazone.

REFERENCE

GOLDING, D. N. (1971), *Postgraduate Medical Journal*, **47**, 611.

IDIOPATHIC HYPOPARATHYROIDISM

This rarely causes a syndrome which may be mistaken for ankylosing spondylitis. There is back pain and stiffness with limitation of spinal movement. This is associated with features of hypocalcaemia, cataracts, fits, tetany, and rashes. Serum calcium is low, phosphates high. XR of the spine show ligamentous calcification as in ankylosing spondylitis. There is soft-tissue calcification and new bone formation around the pelvis and hips, and increased bone density. Sacro-iliac joints are normal.

REFERENCE

JIMENEA, C. V., and others (1971), *Clinical Orthopaedics*, **74**, 84.

IDIOPATHIC STEATORRHOEA

Arthralgia or arthritis is occasional presenting feature of idiopathic steatorrhoea. It typically affects young adults and is easily overlooked since bowel symptoms may be minimal or absent. The pattern of joint involvement is variable with spine, central and peripheral joints sometimes affected. Joints usually appear normal but swelling and effusion occasionally occur. The condition may persist for many years before the diagnosis is made and it may also be episodic. The diagnosis of idiopathic steatorrhoea is confirmed by small bowel biopsy which shows a flat mucosa. Treatment with a gluten-free diet usually leads to a gradual improvement in rheumatic manifestations. Though the condition may bear some clinical resemblance to enteropathic synovitis and ankylosing spondylitis, these conditions do not occur in association with idiopathic steatorrhoea.

INFECTIVE ENDOCARDITIS

A septicaemic illness with infection of heart valves. Musculoskeletal manifestations are of four types:[1,2]
1. Arthralgia or arthritis, described below.
2. Acute febrile lumbago. Episodes of localized pain with muscle spasm and tenderness last for days or weeks, sometimes recurring. Rarely the cervical spine is affected or the whole spine producing a meningitis-like illness.
3. Myalgia again associated with fever, either localized to proximal muscles of the shoulder or pelvic girdle or generalized, bilateral and symmetrical.
4. Pseudohypertrophic osteoarthropathy[3] (rare).

These and other manifestations including renal disease and skin lesions are now believed to be caused by circulating immune complexes.

Incidence

M. = F.
Any age.
25 per cent have joint manifestations; commoner in the elderly.
Usually occurring early in the course of the disease and often a presenting feature.

Joints affected

Usually a few large joints; knees, elbows, ankles and wrists commonest. Occasionally small joints of hands or feet including big toe. Asymmetrical. Occasionally migratory.

Symptoms

Pain, often severe.

Signs

Variable from none to swelling, tenderness, warmth, erythema, and effusion.

Course

Arthritis is episodic. Attacks last 5–15 days and often recur. Responds to antibiotics— no residua. Mortality untreated 100 per cent; treated 30 per cent.

Laboratory

Anaemia, polymorph leucocytosis, and raised E.S.R.
Blood culture positive—*Strep. viridans* in 50 per cent. Repeat again and again if suspicious—many negatives may precede first positive culture. Unusual organisms becoming commoner.
Normal ASO titre. Positive latex test (50 per cent). Hyperglobulinaemia.
Microscopic haematuria (30 per cent).
Albuminuria.

Associations

1. History of pre-existing heart disease (rheumatic, congenital, or arteriosclerotic), recent dental extraction or minor operation, weight loss and fatigue.
2. Fever (95 per cent), characteristically of irregular remittent type with afebrile periods.
3. Cardiac murmurs (95 per cent). Those which appear or change during the course of the disease are especially characteristic.
4. Splenomegaly (40 per cent)—slight.
5. Skin lesions (10 per cent): purpura, petechiae, pustules, painful nodular erythema (Osler's nodes—crops of pea-sized, vivid pink nodules with white centres formed in the skin of the tips of the fingers or toes which disappear within hours or days).
6 Nail lesions; splinter haemorrhages, clubbing.
7. Tenosynovitis rarely.
8. Unusual manifestations: retinal or conjunctival haemorrhage; cerebral 'embolism' causing hemiplegia or chorea.

XR

Joints normal.

INFECTIVE ENDOCARDITIS (*continued*)

Treatment

1. Antibiotics, appropriate to *in vitro* sensitivity of organisms, in doses sufficient to produce bactericidal blood levels, for 6 weeks.
2. Bed rest.
3. Response to analgesic and anti-inflammatory agents disappointing. Absence of response to aspirin in a case of recurrent rheumatic fever should suggest infective endocarditis.

REFERENCES

[1] DESHAYES, P. and others (1974), *Revue du Rhumatisme*, **41**, 135.
[2] MEYERS, O. L. and COMMERFORD, P. J. (1977). *Annals of Rheumatic Diseases*, **36**, 517.
[3] McCORD, M. C., and MOBERLY, J. (1953), *Annals of Internal Medicine*, **39**, 640.

INSTABILITY OF THE PUBIC SYMPHYSIS

A condition described in football players who develop pain in the symphysis pubis, lower abdomen, and groins resembling that of osteitis pubis (*see* p. 88). XR show that when the player stands on one leg, there is movement of one surface of the joint relative to the other. If the symptoms fail to respond to a period of rest and analgesics, arthrodesis of the joint should be carried out.

REFERENCES

The Sunday Times, 13 Feb., 1972.

HARRIS, N. H., and MURRAY, R. O. (1974) *British Medical Journal*, **4**, 211.

INTERMITTENT HYDRARTHROSIS

A rare condition characterized by recurrent joint effusions, usually of the knee, which occur at regular intervals. The condition is usually idiopathic but effusions may rarely recur at regular intervals in rheumatoid arthritis, ankylosing spondylitis, and Reiter's disease. The condition is distinguished from palindromic rheumatism (*see* p. 94) by the regularity of the attacks and by the pattern of joint involvement.

Incidence

M.=F.
Any age, peak 20–50.

Joints affected

Usually one or two joints.
Knees commonest (90 per cent).
65 per cent have involvement only of the knees and of these 60 per cent have bilateral attacks or both knees involved at different times; 40 per cent have only one knee affected.
Occasionally affects elbow or hip (15 per cent cent).
Rarely shoulder, ankle, hands, feet, or temporomandibular joint.
Usually affects the same area in every attack.

Symptoms

Pain, stiffness, swelling.

Signs

Effusion, often large.
Joints are not warm, red, or tender.
Fever occasionally.

Course

Effusion lasts 2–6 days and recurs at regular intervals of 3–30 days (particularly 10, 14, or 21). Periodicity is usually fairly constant in one patient.
The condition continues for years, but 60 per cent have spontaneous remissions lasting up to 10 years.
No deformities.
No tendency to become rheumatoid arthritis.

XR

Normal.
Degenerative changes may appear in long-standing cases.

INTERMITTENT HYDRARTHROSIS (*continued*)

Laboratory

E.S.R. usually normal.
Latex test negative.
Synovial fluid: clear; W.B.C. less than
6000×10^9/dl., predominantly
mononuclear.
No crystals.
Biopsy: non-specific synovitis.

Treatment

1. Analgesics and anti-inflammatory drugs
   when required.
2. Aspiration of fluid.
3. Intra-articular steroids have little or no
   effect.
4. Temporary remissions are sometimes
   induced by gold therapy, radiotherapy, or
   synovectomy. These should be reserved
   for patients who are seriously handicapped
   by the disease.

REFERENCE

MATTINGLY, S. (1957), *British Medical Journal*, **1**, 139.

INTERVERTEBRAL DISC CALCIFICATION IN CHILDREN

A self-limiting syndrome characterized by pain localized to or referred from a segment of the spine, usually cervical, accompanied by radiological evidence of calcification of appropriate intervertebral discs and presumably due to deposition of hydroxyapatite. Because of the marked inflammatory changes that may ensue, a diagnosis of osteomyelitis may be considered.

Incidence

Rare.
Children—average age 7.
M. 2 : 1

Joints affected

Cervical spine commonest (75 per cent).
Occasionally upper dorsal spine (25 per cent).
Rarely lumbar spine.
Usually one site only (95 per cent).
May also affect peripheral joints such as
the shoulder.

Symptoms

Pain in the neck or elsewhere in the spine;
sometimes referred pain.
Stiffness.

Signs

Limitation of movement of affected region.
Local tenderness. Sometimes fever.

Course

Recovers completely within days or weeks.
No sequelae. Occasionally recurrent.

Associations

None.

XR

Calcification of one or occasionally two
intervertebral discs. Usually follows onset
of symptoms, appearing within 2 weeks.
May precede symptoms. Changes may
disappear or persist for many years.

Laboratory

Mild leucocytosis.
Slight elevation of E.S.R.
Otherwise nothing exciting.

Treatment

1. Anti-inflammatory drugs.
2. Immobilization in a collar in the acute
   stage; then exercises to restore movement
   and muscle power.

REFERENCE

EYRING, E. J. and others (1964), *Journal of Bone and Joint Surgery*, **46A**, 1432.

ARTHRITIS AND INTESTINAL BY-PASS FOR OBESITY

About 25 per cent of obese patients treated by either jejunocolostomy or ileocolostomy and 7 per cent of those treated by jejuno-ileostomy develop arthritis or arthralgia. They are mostly young adult females. The small joints of the hands or feet and wrists are commonly affected, sometimes knees, ankles, neck or shoulders. It is equally often symmetrical and asymmetrical, monarticular and polyarticular. The arthritis usually starts suddenly between 6 weeks and 9 months after the by-pass operation. There is pain, sometimes associated with warmth, swelling and tenderness of affected joints. The arthritis often resolves completely within weeks usually in a year but rarely lasts for several years. Associated findings include weight loss, diarrhoea, orthostatic hypertension, gastric ulcer, tetany, renal stone, dehydration, hepatic failure, anaemia and tenosynovitis. E.S.R. may be raised; latex, A.N.F. and L.E. cells are negative. XRs are normal. Synovial biopsy shows non-specific inflammatory changes. Deformities never develop. Treatment: Anti-inflammatory and analgesic drugs—sometimes steroids. Antibiotics may be effective. Closing the by-pass is always effective. In these patients, circulating cryoprotein immune complexes have been demonstrated containing IgG, IgM, IgA and complement. IgG antibody activity was demonstrated by immunofluorescence against two intestinal bacteria, *E. coli* and *B. gracilis*. The implication is that this condition is caused by immune complexes containing bacterial antigens and their antibodies.

REFERENCES

SHAGRIN, J. W., and others (1971), *Annals of Internal Medicine*, **75**, 377.

WANDS, J. R., and others (1976), *New England Journal of Medicine*, **294**, 121.

JACCOUD'S SYNDROME

A very rare sequel of rheumatic fever, usually severe with repeated attacks. The characteristic feature is ulnar deviation at the M.C.P. joints, thought to be due to periarticular fibrosis. This develops after the acute illness and may be analogous to the pathological process which takes place in heart valves.

Incidence

M. = F.
Onset in later childhood or early adult life, months or years after acute rheumatic fever.

Joints affected

M.C.P. joints of hands.
Bilateral and symmetrical.

Symptoms

Stiffness and deformity.
Pain slight or absent.

Signs

Marked ulnar deviation of fingers, mostly the little finger, with flexion of M.C.P. joints and hyperextension of P.I.P. joints.
Function well preserved.
No joint tenderness or swelling, no evidence of active arthritis.

Course

Benign; non-progressive.

Associations

Signs of rheumatic heart disease.

XR

Hook-like erosions may be seen in the metacarpal heads.

Laboratory

Normal E.S.R.
Latex test negative.

Treatment

Not required.

Variant

A similar deformity is an uncommon sequel to S.L.E. (*see* p. 132).

REFERENCE

BYWATERS, E. G. L. (1950), *British Heart Journal*, **12**, 101.

JUMPER'S KNEE (Sinding-Larsen-Johannson's disease; High-jumper's knee; Basket-baller's knee; Volley-baller's knee; Cross-country knee; Place-kicker's knee; High diver's knee; Triple-jumper's knee)

A condition similar to tennis elbow but occurring at the inferior pole of the patella or less commonly the superior pole at the attachment of the patellar tendon. There is pain, local swelling and tenderness, aggravated by exertion. Treatment: Rest; local injection of prednisolone.

JUVENILE CHRONIC ARTHRITIS

A group of diseases of unknown aetiology which begin before the sixteenth birthday. In the past, these diseases have variously been labelled juvenile rheumatoid arthritis and Still's disease, but it is now clear that there are several distinct syndromes. Because it is not always possible to decide in which category a particular patient fits, it is best to make a diagnosis of 'juvenile chronic arthritis (JCA)' and to add the subtype when possible. The disease is subdivided as follows:

A. *Still's disease* (70 per cent of cases); a disease quite unlike rheumatoid arthritis described by G. F. Still in 1897 and characterized by a seronegative arthritis with distinctive and often prominent systemic features such as fever and rash. Three subtypes are described, *Systemic* (25 per cent), *Oligoarticular* (35 per cent) and *Polyarticular* (40 per cent).

In the *Systemic* type, patients present with a high remittent fever, usually a rash, and sometimes other non-articular manifestations such as lymphadenopathy, splenomegaly, hepatomegaly and pericarditis (*see* associations). This type is most often seen in children aged 2–4 with males and females equally affected. Arthritis (or arthralgia) appears within a few months (or occasionally years) of the onset of the disease, is often a minor feature of the illness and is occasionally absent. It may affect one or many joints and is of variable severity. About 25 per cent of these patients develop a severe progressive arthritis.
In the other types, arthritis is the most prominent feature though systemic manifestations like fever and rash may also be present.

The *Oligoarticular* type affects females twice as often as males and usually starts before age 5. Patients have up to 4 joints involved, particularly large joints such as the knees. Hips, ankles, elbows and occasionally small joints of the hands or feet may be affected. In these patients there is a high incidence of chronic iritis (30 per cent). Antinuclear factor is positive in 80 per cent of patients with iritis and provides a useful warning. Because the iritis is often symptomless at onset and leads to blindness if untreated, regular screening with slit-lamp examination is essential.

The *Polyarticular* Type is the commonest variety and arthritis is the most important feature. It usually begins before age 5 and affects females twice as often as males. There is an acute or insidious onset of arthritis, usually bilateral and symmetrical but affecting knees, wrists, ankles and elbows. The small joints of the hands and feet are affected less often than in rheumatoid arthritis and distal interphalangeal joint involvement may be prominent. The neck, hips and temporomandibular joints may be affected. Joint pain is often mild. Patients may complain of swelling, stiffness or difficulty with walking or other functions. Affected joints are usually swollen, warm and tender with effusion and limitation of movement.

Course
Chronic with remissions and relapses. Most cases have a good prognosis. 80 per cent are eventually able to lead a normal life; 20 per cent disabled to a variable extent; 8 per cent die of infection or amyloidosis. In most cases the activity settles within a few years. A few continue into adult life and may develop severe destructive joint changes, ankylosis and deformities. About 20 per cent of cases have one episode lasting up to 2 years and recover without any sequelae. About 55 per cent have multiple episodes lasting weeks or months with inactive periods between and eventual complete remission. 25 per cent become chronic with variable activity. Premature fusion of epiphyses may lead to stunting of growth (dwarfism) or local abnormalities such as micrognathism. Best prognosis with acute onset; worst when insidious.

JUVENILE CHRONIC ARTHRITIS (*continued*)

Associations
1. Fever (20 per cent). Remittent, with evening peaks up to 40 °C. Often suggests the possibility of sepsis.
2. Rash (45 per cent): patches of erythema on the trunk or limbs, often seen towards the end of the day and brought out by a hot bath. No itching in 95 per cent but when present, it may be intense. Koebner phenomenon may occur: erythema appears within a few minutes of rubbing or scratching the skin.
3. Splenomegaly (35 per cent).
4. Lymphadenopathy (45 per cent).
5. Pericarditis (10 per cent). Rarely myocarditis in patients with severe systemic disease.
6. Iritis (10 per cent of all cases but 30 per cent of oligoarticular type) associated with positive A.N.F. Often symptomless. May lead to synechiae, band keratopathy, glaucoma and cataract.
7. Nodules (5 per cent). Histology more often resembles that of the rheumatic fever nodule than the rheumatoid nodule.
   Less common manifestations include:
8. Abdominal pain due to mesenteric adenitis or peritonitis.
9. Drowsiness, irritability, fits and meningism in the acute stage.

XR
Often normal, especially in the early stages. Later there may be:
1. Periarticular osteoporosis
2. Periosteal proliferation.
3. Enlargement and premature fusion of epiphyses, leading to growth disturbances, e.g. short phalanges.
4. Erosions and loss of joint space are late and unusual.
5. Bony fusion of joints may result, particularly in the carpus and cervical spine.
6. Atlanto-axial subluxation is rare.

Laboratory
Anaemia and raised E.S.R. proportional to activity. Leucocytosis common with systemic disease (50 per cent): usually 15–30,000 but occasionally up to $80,000 \times 10^9$ cells/dl. Latex test usually negative. A.N.F. positive in 30 per cent: Strong association with iritis. Synovial fluid: inflammatory. Mainly polymorphs.

Management
1. *Non-steroidal anti-inflammatory drugs.* Aspirin remains first choice. Use full anti-inflammatory dose (80 mg./kg./day in 4–6 divided doses) and check plasma levels (should be 20–30 mg./dl.). Soluble variety or sophisticated preparations such as aloxiprin, usually preferred. Alternatives include ibuprofen (up to 40 mg./kg./day) and other propionic acid derivatives. Indomethacin at night (2.5 mg./kg.) for morning stiffness. Avoid phenylbutazone.
2. *Rest.* Bed rest for acutely ill child. Splint affected joints but ensure maintenance of full range of movement and muscle power with daily physiotherapy.
3. *Joint protection.* Splints and exercises to prevent deformity and loss of movement of affected joints. Hydrotherapy often useful for diseases of weight-bearing joints. Exercises such as prone lying to prevent flexion deformity of hip.
4. *Gold or penicillamine* for patients with progressive or uncontrolled disease despite adequate anti-inflammatory therapy, rest etc.
   Gold: 1 mg./kg. I.M. weekly until response, then maintenance doses as in adults.
   Pencillamine: Start with 25 or 50 mg. daily and increase monthly. Usual maintenance dose is 200–500 mg. daily.
5. *Regular 6-monthly slit lamp examination* for iritis. Local steroids and atropine if it occurs.
6. *Ensure continued education* and as normal a life-style as possible. Encourage swimming and gentle pursuits.
7. *Avoid contact sports* like football while joints are active.
8. *Avoid systemic corticosteroids.* When essential, use alternate day prednisolone or ACTH to preserve growth.
9. *Surgery* for the joint which is irreversibly damaged.
10. *Parental involvement* essential in programme of drug administration and joint protection and maintenance.

Still's disease occasionally occurs in adults[4] after age 16, just as rheumatoid arthritis occasionally occurs before. It begins up to the age of 35 and is commoner in females. Arthritis is usually recurrent with episodes lasting weeks or months. Knees, wrists and small joints of the hands are the commonest affected joints. As in children distal interphalangeal joint involvement may be prominent. Ankles, shoulders, neck and occasionally hips may also be affected. In most cases the number of joints involved is fewer than in adult rheumatoid arthritis, most cases having 2 or 3 sites affected. Arthritis is usually bilateral. In most cases the arthritis resolves without residua even though it may be recurrent. A few develop ankylosis of joints in the wrist or neck particularly and occasionally the arthritis is chronic, destructive and eventually disabling. Systemic features are prominent, in particular fever, rash, pericarditis, pleurisy and splenomegaly. Fever is usually a prominent feature and is remittent often suggesting the possibility of sepsis. Rheumatoid subcutaneous nodules are not found. XR is often normal but erosions are present in severe cases and mild sacroiliac changes (sclerosis of joint margins) may be seen. ESR may be raised but the latex test and ANF are negative. Synovial biopsy shows mild non-specific inflammatory changes. Treatment: anti-inflammatory drugs.

B. *Juvenile Rheumatoid Arthritis* (15 per cent of cases). These patients tend to be female and the disease starts most often between the ages of 12 and 15. The pattern of joint involvement resembles that of adult rheumatoid arthritis (p. 114) with early and prominent involvement of the small joints of the hands—many joints are affected in a bilateral symmetrical distribution. There is usually persistent activity and untreated, the disease is progressive and leads to joint destruction. Rheumatoid factor is found in 70 per cent of cases and erosions are commonly seen in X-rays of the hands and feet. Systemic features of Still's disease such as fever and rash are not seen but nodules occur occasionally. Treatment with gold or penicillamine is often required and often successful in these patients and should be used if anti-inflammatory therapy fails to control the disease.

C. *Ankylosing Spondylitis and Polyarthritis associated with Sacroiliitis and HLA B27* (15 per cent of cases). These patients tend to be male with disease starting most often between the ages of 9 and 12. The lower limb is predominantly involved, particularly knees, ankles and feet. About half of these patients develop ankylosing spondylitis—the remainder develop sacroiliitis without evidence of spinal involvement. Acute iritis may occur in the group and HLA B27 is almost always present. A family history of ankylosing spondylitis is sometimes helpful in diagnosis.

Differential Diagnosis of Arthritis in Children
The range of disorders which must be considered is a little different in children and includes:
1. Juvenile chronic arthritis of various types (*above*).
2. Rheumatic fever (p. 113).
3. Henoch-Schönlein disease (p. 44).
4. Acute leukaemia (p. 67).
5. Systemic lupus erythematosus (p. 132). 15 per cent of cases occur in children.
6. Dermatomyositis (p. 102) and scleroderma (p. 121).
7. Psoriatic arthropathy (p. 105).
8. Traumatic arthritis (p. 142).
9. Infections: Septic arthritis, tuberculosis, rubella, mumps etc.
10. Perthes' disease (p. 96).
11. Transient synovitis of the hip (p. 141).
12. Enteropathic synovitis (p. 28).
13. Post-dysenteric Reiter's disease (p. 110).
14. Familial Mediterranean Fever (p. 32).
15. Hypogammaglobulinaemia.
16. 'Growing pains'—possibly psychogenic and not accompanied by swelling or other objective abnormalities of joints.
17. Erythema nodosum (p. 31).
18. Sickle-cell disease (p. 126).
19. Clutton's joints (p. 20).
20. Plant thorn synovitis (p. 98).

REFERENCES

[1] ANSELL, B. M., and BYWATERS, E. G. L. (1959), *Bulletin on Rheumatic Diseases*, 26, 1850.

[2] BYWATERS, E. G. L. (1967), *Annals of Rheumatic Diseases*, 26, 185.

[3] CALABRO, J. J. and others (1976), *Seminars in Arthritis and Rheumatism*, 5, 257.

[4] BYWATERS, E. G. L. (1971), *Annals of Rheumatic Diseases*, 30, 121.

[5] ANSELL, B. M., and HALL, M. A. (1976), *Reports on Rheumatic Diseases*, No. 59. London: Arthritis and Rheumatism Council.

KASHIN-BECK DISEASE (Urov Disease; Osteoarthritis Deformans)

A degenerative arthropathy, endemic in Eastern Siberia, Northern China, and Northern Korea, due to infection of cereal grain in these areas with the fungus *Fusaria sporotrichiella*. The incidence of the disease is declining with the elimination of infected grain.

Incidence

M. = F.
Onset in children and young adults.

Joints affected

Fingers commonest; also wrists, ankles, knees, hips, and later spine.
Bilateral and symmetrical.

Symptoms

Insidious onset of pain, often mild, swelling, and stiffness; worst after activity.

Signs

Bony swelling, crepitus, limitation of movement.
No inflammatory changes or effusion.
Later deformities and shortening of fingers (arthritis mutilans) and limbs.

Course

Chronic, with slow progress to complete disability.

Associations

No systemic features.

XR

Degenerative changes: loss of joint space, sclerosis, and cysts.
Later destruction of bone, particularly phalanges.

Laboratory

Normal E.S.R.
Negative latex test.

Treatment

Analgesics.

REFERENCE

NESTEROV, A. I. (1964), *Arthritis and Rheumatism*, 7, 29.

KNUCKLE-PAD SYNDROME

Knobbly knuckles (k.k. syndrome or Garrod's fatty pads), characterized by the development of fleshy pads over the dorsum of the proximal interphalangeal joint of the fingers. They appear at any age in either sex. Patients with this harmless condition often complain of joint swelling and fear that they have rheumatoid arthritis. Occasionally there is pain and tenderness, but the joint itself is clinically and radiologically normal. The syndrome is often associated with Dupuytren's contracture, or a family history of Dupuytren's contracture. Reassurance is usually sufficient therapy.

REFERENCE

GARROD, A. E. (1904), *British Medical Journal*, 2, 8.

LEPROSY

Infection with *Mycobacterium leprae* found in tropical Africa and Asia, South America, and the Far East. The disease is manifest predominantly as chronic skin lesions, with intermittent febrile 'reactions'. Arthritis is of two types:
1. *Acute polyarthritis* associated with reactions, particularly erythema nodosum leprosum, described below.[1]
2. *Neuropathic arthropathy* (*see* p. 83), due to chronic peripheral neuropathy and affecting distal joints of the hands or hands and feet, spreading proximally. This is associated with trophic ulceration, destruction of bone, and sometimes complete loss of fingers, toes, hands, and feet.[2]

Incidence
M. 10 : 1.
Peak in young adults.
5 per cent have episodes of arthritis at some time.
Arthritis occurs after several years of disease, associated with exacerbation of skin lesions and often while on sulphone therapy.

Joints affected
P.I.P. and M.C.P. joints, wrists, knees, and ankles commonest.
Others occasionally. Bilateral and symmetrical, resembling rheumatoid arthritis.

Symptoms
Acute onset of pain and stiffness.

Signs
Joints are swollen and tender.
Effusion usual.
Fever.

Course
Arthritis usually resolves within a few weeks with resolution of other features of the 'reaction'; occasionally lasts up to 1 year. No residua.
May recur with subsequent reactions.

Associations
1. Erythema nodosum leprosum; erythematous nodules appear on the limbs.
2. Skin lesions of lepromatous leprosy; less commonly dimorphous or tuberculoid type.
3. Palpable tender peripheral nerves; sensory peripheral neuropathy.
4. Iritis, orchitis, or lymphadenopathy.

XR
Usually normal.
May show periarticular porosis.

Laboratory
Raised E.S.R.
Positive latex test and L.E. cells in about 50 per cent.
Synovial fluid: non-inflammatory; sterile on culture.
Skin biopsy shows acid-fast bacilli in lepromatous lesions.

Treatment
1. Clofazimine 100 mg. t.d.s.
2. Salicylates as required.
3. Long-term dapsone (minimum 2 years).
4. Short course of steroids rarely required for severe reactions.

REFERENCES

[1] KARAT, A. B. A., and others (1967), *British Medical Journal*, 3, 770.

[2] LELE, R. D., and others (1965), *Journal of the Association of Physicians of India*, 13, 275.

LÉRI'S PLEONOSTEOSIS

A rare hereditary disorder characterized by contractures of the fingers, due to fibrous contraction of the capsular ligaments of the small joints, and associated with various other abnormalities.

Incidence

M. = F.
Onset in early childhood.
F.H. usual.

Joints affected

Hands and feet usually.
Others rare.
Bilateral and symmetrical.

Symptoms

Pain in hands and feet, associated with increasing contractures of fingers and toes.

Signs

Flexion deformities of fingers and toes; rarely also elbows.
Thumbs and great toes are characteristically broad.
Limitation of movement of fingers, toes, and rarely also hips, knees, shoulders, elbows, and wrists.

Course

Slow progressive increase in contracture.

Associations

1. Shortness of stature (common).
2. Mongoloid facies (common).
3. Other joint abnormalities (coxa vara or genu valgum).
4. Carpal tunnel syndrome (occasionally).
5. Intellectual impairment (rare).

XR

Broad metacarpals, metatarsals, and phalanges.
No joint changes.

Laboratory

Unhelpful.

Treatment

1. Analgesics if required.
2. Maintain mobility with exercises.
3. Surgical correction of contractures occasionally required.

REFERENCE

WATSON-JONES, R. (1949), *Journal of Bone and Joint Surgery*, **31B**, 560.

ACUTE LEUKAEMIA

A neoplastic condition in which there is proliferation of primitive white blood-cells, classified according to the type of cell (myeloblastic, lymphoblastic, monocytic, and undifferentiated). Arthritis is due either to haemorrhage in or around the joint or to leukaemic infiltration of bone or soft tissues. Acute leukaemia may also be associated with secondary gout (*see* p. 39), or opportunistic infection which may cause septic arthritis (*see* p. 123). Aspiration is essential for persistent acute arthritis which fails to respond to salicylates.

Incidence

M. = F.
15 per cent of children and 5 per cent of adults have arthritis; commonest with lymphoblastic type.
Arthritis may precede other manifestations by up to 2 years.

Joints affected

Lower limb in 90 per cent; upper limb in 40 per cent.
Spine and knee commonest; also hips, feet, ankles, shoulders, elbows, and hands.
Commonly bilateral and symmetrical.
10 per cent monarticular; 40 per cent migratory.

Symptoms

Pain is usually severe; sudden or insidious onset.
Diffuse 'boring' pain in spine and limb bones is characteristic.

Signs

Swelling, warmth, erythema, and marked tenderness.
Fever common.

Course

Arthritis improves with remission of leukaemia; otherwise chronic with periods of improvement, followed by exacerbation.

Associations

30 per cent have no physical findings other than arthritis.
70 per cent have pallor sometimes with splenomegaly (50 per cent), hepatomegaly (40 per cent), lymphadenopathy (40 per cent), or purpura (20 per cent).

XR

40 per cent normal.
Other findings are:
1. Periarticular osteoporosis.
2. Periosteal elevation.
3. Osteolytic lesions.

Laboratory

Diagnosis is made by finding large numbers of 'blast' cells in a peripheral blood-film; 15 per cent have normal film early in the course of the disease; if suspicious ask for bone-marrow examination.
Total W.B.C. often normal.
Anaemia common.
Latex test occasionally positive.
Hyperuricaemia may be found.

Treatment

1. Salicylates.
2. Specific antileukaemic therapy—combinations of steroids and cytotoxic drugs to induce remission.

REFERENCE

SILVERSTEIN, M. N., and KELLY, P. J. (1963), *Annals of Internal Medicine*, **59**, 637.

CHRONIC LEUKAEMIA

A malignant proliferation of the lymphocyte (lymphocytic) or polymorph (myeloid) precursors, characterized by the presence of large numbers of lymphocytes or myelocytes in circulating blood and in certain tissues. Arthritis is probably due to infiltration of such cells in the synovium. There is also a high incidence of secondary gout, especially during treatment.

Incidence

M. = F.
Adults; peak age 60.
12 per cent have arthritis.
Commonest during the course of the disease (50 per cent) but may precede other manifestations by an average of 2 years (25 per cent), or occur at the onset of the disease (25 per cent).

Joints affected

Knees commonest (60 per cent).
Occasionally shoulders, hips, elbows, small joints of hands or feet, wrists, and ankles.
70 per cent are eventually symmetrical; 30 per cent migratory; 20 per cent monarticular.

Symptoms

Pain and swelling.

Signs

Affected joints are usually warm, red, and swollen.

Course

Attacks of arthritis last up to 4 weeks and disappear with response to treatment of leukaemia. Recurrence occasional (20 per cent).
Untreated patients survive for about 3 years, but up to 10 or longer with the benign lymphatic type in the elderly. Death is due either to acute blastic phase or anaemia due to bone-marrow failure.

Associations

1. Insidious onset of fatigue and pallor due to anaemia.
2. Hepatosplenomegaly.
3. Lymphadenopathy, particularly with lymphatic type.
4. Skin lesions with lymphatic type.
5. Bruising and bleeding.
6. Infections.

XR

Usually normal. Sometimes porosis of surrounding bone.

Laboratory

W.B.C. up to 500,000 $\times$ 10^9/dl. lymphocytes or myelocytes predominate.
Bone-marrow confirms.
Latex test or A.N.F. occasionally positive (15 per cent).
Hyperuricaemia (15 per cent).
Synovial fluid: inflammatory;
W.B.C. about 5000 $\times$ 10^9/dl., mainly polymorphs but not abnormal.

Treatment

1. Aspirin, phenylbutazone, or indomethacin.
2. Specific treatment for leukaemia with cytotoxic drugs and radiotherapy; blood transfusion if necessary.

REFERENCE

SPILBERG, I., and MAYER, G. T. (1972), *Arthritis and Rheumatism*, **15**, 12.

LONG-LEG ARTHROPATHY

Arises in the knee of the longer leg of patients who continue to walk with inequality of leg length for many years. Such patients walk with the longer leg flexed and externally rotated at the hip and flexed at the knee so that there is a repeated valgus strain. Osteoarthritis develops causing pain, swelling, and stiffness. *Moral*: inequality of leg length should be corrected by raising the height of one shoe. This is particularly important in patients who already have disease of the knees and develop shortening of one limb, e.g., in rheumatoid arthritis.

REFERENCE

DIXON, A. ST. J., and CAMPBELL-SMITH, S. (1969), *Annals of the Rheumatic Diseases*, **28**, 359.

LYME ARTHRITIS

Named after the part of East Connecticut, U.S.A. where it occurs; this is an epidemic asymmetrical oligoarthritis characterized by recurrent brief attacks of joint pain and swelling, possibly caused by an arthropod-transmitted infection. The disease is most likely to be mistaken for juvenile chronic arthritis.

Incidence
Children (80 per cent) and young adults. Mean age 11 (2–45).
M. = F.
Peak incidence in summer.
Prevalence: 0·4 per cent in the Lyme area and up to 1 per cent in Lyme itself (much commoner than juvenile chronic arthritis).

Joints affected
About 3 joints in each attack; asymmetrical. Large joints—knees commonest (85 per cent). Ankle, wrist, shoulder, temporomandibular joint, hip or elbow in 5–10 per cent of attacks. Pain in hands or feet in about 10 per cent.

Symptoms
Sudden onset of swelling, often with pain in knee or other large joints—monarticular onset in 70 per cent.

Signs
Marked swelling with effusion, tenderness, and sometimes, warmth.

Course
Attacks last on average one week but rarely up to 6 months. Recurrence in 70 per cent, usually brief and lasting about one week. Average 2 months between attacks but up to 23 months. Average patient has 3 recurrences (2–10). Complete remission between attacks and no permanent sequelae.

Associations
1. Erythema chronicum migrans (25 per cent), an erythematous papule usually on an extremity which expands to an annular lesion up to 50 cm. in diameter. Occasionally multiple. Starts on average 4 weeks before arthritis (1–24 weeks) and lasts for days or weeks. Commoner in adults than children.
2. Fever (60 per cent), malaise, fatigue, headache, myalgia and occasionally a maculopapular rash.

XR
Normal.

Laboratory
Normal blood count.
E.S.R. slightly raised.
Synovial fluid: inflammatory: W.B.C. up to $100,000 \times 10^9$/dl. (mean 26,000), mainly polymorphs.
Latex and A.N.F. negative. Low C3 in some patients.
Synovial biopsy: hypertrophy, vascular proliferation and infiltration with lymphocytes and plasma cells. No organism yet identified.

Treatment
Symptomatic: aspirin or other anti-inflammatory drugs.

REFERENCE

STEERE, A. C. and others (1977), *Arthritis and Rheumatism*, **20**, 7.

LYMPHOEDEMA PRAECOX

Causes painless swelling of the ankle or foot and may be confused with arthritis. It usually begins at about the time of puberty, and affects girls predominantly. The oedema is at first aggravated by activity and relieved by rest but progresses slowly to chronic lymphoedema of the limb.

LYMPHOGRANULOMA VENEREUM

A venereal disease caused by a large virus. After an incubation period of 1–4 weeks, a small ulcer forms on the external genitalia or in the rectum with inguinal lymphadenopathy, fever, and malaise. 5 per cent of patients have arthralgia at this stage. The lymph-nodes may later break down forming sinuses. Involvement of the rectum causes proctitis with a purulent discharge. Chronic disease leads to rectal stricture, lymphatic obstruction and oedema, and perineal fistulae.

Incidence

M. = F.
Age 15–40; particularly sexually promiscuous. Arthritis at any stage; commoner with chronic proctitis.

Joints affected

Polyarticular.
Ankles, hips, elbows, and wrists commonest.
Usually asymmetrical.
Rarely migratory.

Symptoms

Pain and swelling.

Signs

Joints are red, warm, and tender with effusion.
Fever common.

Course

Arthritis lasts for 1–2 weeks, then resolves completely, but tends to recur at irregular intervals if disease continues.
Complete cure with early antibiotic therapy.

Associations

1. Skin lesions common: generalized pustular eruption, erythema nodosum or erythema multiforme.
2. Tenosynovitis (rare).
3. Inguinal lymphadenopathy and signs of pelvic disease.

XR

Normal.

Laboratory

Anaemia, leucocytosis, and raised E.S.R.
Diagnosis confirmed by Frei test (intra-dermal injection of killed virus suspension), complement-fixation test, or gland biopsy.
Synovial fluid: non-inflammatory;
W.B.C. less than $10,000 \times 10^9$/dl.

Treatment

1. Tetracycline 250 mg. q.d.s. for 10 days.
2. Analgesics and anti-inflammatory drugs.

Variants

Very rarely arthritis of one hip occurs, resembling septic arthritis, and leading to bone destruction.

REFERENCE

HICKAM, J. B. (1945), *Archives of Dermatology and Syphilology*, **51**, 330.

MACRODYSTROPHIA LIPOMATOSA

A rare, non-familial condition characterized by lipomatous enlargement of one or more fingers, and a severe degenerative arthropathy of the metacarpophalangeal and interphalangeal joints of affected fingers. Patients present with pain and swelling of the fingers; a lipoma may press on the median nerve causing carpal tunnel syndrome. Examination reveals soft-tissue swelling of the affected fingers which may be double the size of adjacent normal fingers. The condition is slowly progressive and leads eventually to ankylosis and deformities. XR show enlargement of bones and huge osteophytes around the joints. Treatment: Analgesics.

REFERENCE

RANAWAT, C. S., and others (1968), *Journal of Bone and Joint Surgery*, **50A**, 1242.

MALIGNANT DISEASE AND ARTHRITIS

Arthritis is one of the many ways in which malignant disease may present and the diagnosis is therefore of great importance. Arthritis associated with malignant disease may be of the following types.

1. *Pseudohypertrophic Osteoarthropathy* (*see* p. 104) occurs particularly with pulmonary, pleural, or diaphragmatic tumours; rarely upper gastro-intestinal or cardiac tumours.

2. *Secondary Gout* (*see* p. 39) is a particular feature of the leukaemias, lymphomas, and multiple myeloma. It also occurs with disseminated malignancy particularly during treatment with cytotoxic drugs. Allopurinol provides effective prophylaxis in these conditions.

3. *Skeletal Metastases* cause arthritis when bone adjacent to a joint is involved. This is usually monarticular and X-rays should suggest the correct diagnosis.

4. *Acute Leukaemia* (*see* p. 67) is frequently associated with arthritis, especially in children.

5. *Chronic Leukaemia* (*see* p. 68) also causes arthritis.

6. *Multiple Myeloma* (*see* p. 81) is usually accompanied by back pain but may also cause peripheral arthritis either associated with deposits in bone or amyloidosis (*see* p. 5).

7. *Carcinoma Arthritis* (*see* p. 16) is a condition resembling rheumatoid arthritis which is associated with various malignancies and is not due to metastases in bones or joints.

8. *Dermatomyositis* and, less commonly, *Polymyositis* (*see* p. 102) may be manifestations of malignant disease, particularly carcinoma of the lung, ovary, breast, and stomach; this should be considered especially in adults over 40 and when the condition fails to respond to steroids.

9. *Pyrophosphate Arthropathy* (*see* p. 108) may occur in any condition in which there is hypercalcaemia including malignancy either with or without skeletal metastases.

10. A syndrome resembling *Polymyalgia rheumatica* (*see* p. 101) is occasionally associated with malignant disease, particularly of the bronchus or breast.

11. *Systemic Lupus Erythematosus* (*see* p. 132) is very rarely a manifestation of malignancy.

12. *Opportunistic Infection* may occur in malignant conditions either with general debility or associated with depression of antibody formation as in multiple myeloma or neutropenia as in leukaemias. The manifestations are those of septic arthritis (*see* p. 123) but the organism may be unusual; in these circumstances organisms which are not usually pathogenic may be found.

13. *Lymphomas* cause arthritis by skeletal invasion which is common; they also cause secondary gout, pseudohypertrophic osteoarthropathy, and carcinoma polyarthritis. There is an association between lymphoma and Sjögren's syndrome (dry eyes and dry mouth with rheumatoid arthritis).

14. *Primary Joint Tumours:* Synovioma (*see* p. 129) etc.

15. *Pancreatic Carcinoma* (*see* p. 95) may be associated with subcutaneous nodules and arthritis.

16. *Carcinoid Syndrome* (*see* p. 16) is rarely associated with arthritis.

17. *Erythema Nodosum* and arthritis (*see* p. 31) may be caused by some malignant conditions.

18. *Referred Pain* may suggest joint disease—in particular pain in the shoulder may be the first symptom of bronchial carcinoma.

REFERENCE

CALABRO, J. J. (1967), *Arthritis and Rheumatism*, **10**, 553.

MELIOIDOSIS

Infection with *Pseudomonas pseudomallei*, endemic in South-east Asia. The acute form of the disease is a septicaemic illness with high fever, often fatal. In the chronic form, which may present many years after the patient has left the endemic area, there is pneumonia with metastatic abscess formation in the skin, bones, and viscera. Arthritis occurs in about 2 per cent of cases, particularly in young adult males. It is usually monarticular and most commonly affects the knee. The diagnosis is confirmed by culturing the organism from joint fluid which is turbid with a predominantly polymorph leucocytosis. Treatment: Combined antibiotic therapy, depending on *in vitro* sensitivities, e.g., chloramphenicol, tetracycline, and a sulphonamide.

REFERENCE

DIAMOND, H. S., and PASTORE, R. (1967), *Arthritis and Rheumatism*, **10**, 459.

MELORHEOSTOSIS

A rare, non-hereditary disorder characterized by localized hyperostosis of long bones.

Incidence

M. = F.
Any age; peak in childhood.

Joints affected

Usually one or two joints of one limb.
Lower limb commonly involved: knee, hip, ankle, or foot.
Asymmetrical.

Symptoms

1. Insidious onset of pain and stiffness.
2. Deformities.

Signs

Joints show restriction of movement and there are episodes of warmth and swelling in the active phase.
Deformities are common: limb often short, rarely long; curvature; flexion contracture.

Course

Progresses for a few years then remains static.
Joint pains continue but not usually severe.
Disability unusual.
Osteoarthritis may occur in deformed joints.

Associations

1. Skin over affected areas may be tight, smooth, and shiny, resembling scleroderma.
2. Soft-tissue contractures are common, e.g., palmar or plantar fascial thickening and finger contracture; over-riding toes.

XR

Irregular dense radio-opacity in the line of affected long bones, may extend into pelvis, tarsus, or carpus.
Patchy hyperostosis in epiphyses and carpal or tarsal bones.
Appearance said to resemble wax dripping down a candle.

Laboratory

No abnormality.

Treatment

1. Analgesics.
2. Prevention and correction of deformity with splints, braces, and surgery.

REFERENCE

CAMPBELL, C. J., and others (1968), *Journal of Bone and Joint Surgery*, **50A**, 1281.

MENINGOCOCCAL INFECTION

A disease which is usually sporadic and uncommon but with major epidemics, often in time of war. It affects children and young adults and the most common clinical syndrome is meningitis which may be accompanied by purpura. Less commonly there is fulminating septicaemia with purpura, often fatal, or a chronic septicaemia. Arthritis may be due to infection of the joint but is probably more often due to immune complex disease—complexes of IgM, C3 and meningococcal antigen have been demonstrated. Septic arthritis occurs early during the septicaemic phase and resembles that of other infections. Arthralgia is common in early meningococcal disease and arthritis is a feature of chronic meningococcal septicaemia.

Incidence
6 per cent of patients with meningococcal meningitis have arthritis—commoner in adults (30 per cent over age 30).
M. = F.
Peak incidence 2–6 days after onset of symptoms, often when the patient is on antibiotics and neurological signs are diminishing. May be up to 12 days after onset.

Joints affected
Polyarticular in 60 per cent.
Knee (60 per cent) and wrist (60 per cent) commonest.
Elbow (40 per cent) ankle (35 per cent) fingers (20 per cent) hip (10 per cent)—rarely shoulders or toes.

Symptoms and Signs
When arthritis develops early in the course of the disease, severe pain with no signs is characteristic. When it develops later, painless effusions are characteristic.

Course
Arthritis usually settles within days or weeks. No residua except in septic type.

Associations
1. Vasculitic skin lesions or purpura.
2. Episcleritis.
3. Mild proteinuria.

XR
Normal.

Laboratory
Synovial fluid: W.B.C. about $40,000 \times 10^9$/dl. (up to 100,000)—mainly polymorphs. Often sterile on culture.
Synovial biopsy: inflammatory changes with monocytes and polymorphs.
Diagnosis of meningococcal infection is made by culturing the organism from blood, C.S.F. etc.

Treatment
Penicillin and sulphadiazine for meningococcal infection.
Symptomatic therapy for arthritis unless septic.

REFERENCE

GREENWOOD, B. M., and WHITTLE, H. C. (1976), The pathogenesis of meningococcal arthritis. In: *Infection and Immunology in the Rheumatic Diseases*, Oxford: Blackwell.

MENINGOCOCCAL INFECTION (*continued*)

Chronic Type associated with chronic meningococcal septicaemia.

Incidence
Muscle and joint pains occur in all cases, arthritis in 50 per cent.

Joints affected
Polyarticular.
Knees commonest.
Often other large joints.
Rarely small joints of hands.
Migratory, often asymmetrical.

Symptoms
Sudden or gradual onset of pain in joints and muscles.

Signs
Variable degree of warmth, erythema, tenderness, and effusion.
Fever usual.

Course
Untreated it may last for weeks or months with episodes of fever before metastatic infection (usually meningitis) appears.
Complete resolution without sequelae follows treatment.

Associations
Crops of skin lesions, often sparse, which may be:
1. Pink macules, papules, or nodules, often painful or tender, up to 3 cm. diameter usually on the limbs or back.
2. Petechiae.
3. Tender subcutaneous nodules on the fronts of the legs.
Spleen not usually palpable.

XR
Normal

Laboratory
W.B.C. normal or slightly raised.
Blood-culture required to make the diagnosis; repeat again and again if suspicious.

Treatment
Penicillin and sulphadiazine.

REFERENCE

COPEMAN, W. S. C. (1942), *British Medical Journal*, **1**, 760.

MIXED CONNECTIVE-TISSUE DISEASE

A variant of Systemic Lupus Erythematosus in which clinical features of S.L.E. (p. 132) polymyositis (p. 102) and scleroderma (p. 121) coexist in the same patient. It is worth distinguishing from S.L.E. because it responds well to steroids, pursues a benign course and has an excellent prognosis. It also has distinct serological characteristics.

Incidence
Much less common than S.L.E.
F5 : 1.
Onset in young adults.

Clinical features
S.L.E.-like
Arthritis or arthralgia identical to that of S.L.E. (95 per cent) but renal disease in only 10 per cent and serious C.N.S. disease in only 5 per cent. Other features of S.L.E. (fever, serositis, lung involvement, lymphadenopathy, splenomegaly, erythematous rashes) may occur. Some C.N.S. manifestations in 50 per cent including headache with abnormal C.S.F. resembling aseptic meningitis, peripheral neuropathy, psychiatric disturbance, fits.

Polymyositis-like
Proximal muscle weakness, wasting and pain (60 per cent). Occasionally dusky red rash over eyelids and small joints.

Scleroderma-like
Raynaud's phenomenon (85 per cent).
Puffy hands (75 per cent).
Abnormal oesophageal mobility (65 per cent).
Serious systemic complications of scleroderma are unusual.

Laboratory
Anaemia and leucopenia (50 per cent).
E.S.R. raised.
A.N.F. always positive. Speckled pattern.
DNA binding normal.
E.N.A. antibodies positive—
    anti-R.N.P. positive.
    anti-SM negative.
L.E. cells: 20 per cent.
Latex test often positive.
Complement normal.
Hypergammaglobulinaemia common (80 per cent).
Muscle enzymes (creatine phosphokinase) raised with active muscle disease.

XR
Normal

Treatment
Corticosteroids. Small doses (prednisolone 5–10 mg.). Use smallest possible dose and stop when no longer required.

Course
Usually benign. 5-year survival: 95 per cent
Responds well to steroids, except Raynaud's phenomenon.

REFERENCES

SHARP, G. C., and others (1972), *American Journal of Medicine*, **52**, 148.

PARKER, M. D. (1973), *Journal of Laboratory and Clinical Medicine*, **82**, 769.

MORQUIO-BRAILSFORD SYNDROME

Type IV mucopolysaccharidosis (*see* p. 78). A rare congenital disorder inherited as an autosomal recessive. Skeletal deformities appear in early childhood. Most cases eventually develop corneal and cardiac abnormalities.

Incidence
M. = F.
Onset at age 1–10.

Joints affected
Every joint may be affected in a severe case. Usually spine, hips, and knees.
D.I.P. joints involved as well as P.I.P. and M.C.P. joints.
Bilateral and symmetrical.

Symptoms
Joint swelling and stiffness.
Later deformities.
No pain.

Signs
1. Bony swelling of joints; limitation of movement; flexion deformities.
2. Severe kyphosis leads to characteristic crouching stance with head pushed forwards. Stature reduced.
3. There may be hypermobility of some joints, e.g., wrists and hands.
4. Other skeletal deformities include genu valgum, short neck, and pigeon chest.

Course
Many die before age 20 from respiratory or cardiac failure.
Mild cases survive to adult life, but are usually severely disabled as a result of skeletal deformities.

Associations
1. Dwarfism.
2. Corneal opacity appearing in adolescence.
3. Aortic valve disease.
4. Characteristic facies (wide mouth, prominent maxilla).
5. Spastic paraplegia or quadriplegia with respiratory failure may result from cord compression. Atlanto-axial subluxation is a risk particularly with hyperextension of the cervical spine at anaesthesia.
6. Slight hepatosplenomegaly.

XR
1. Osteoporosis.
2. Flat wedge-shaped vertebrae with anterior 'beaks'.
3. Enlarged irregular epiphysis and later distortion of bone ends.

Laboratory
Increased urinary keratosulphate.
Normal E.S.R.
Negative latex test.

Treatment
Maintain mobility as far as possible.

REFERENCES

ELLMAN, P. (1949), *Annals of the Rheumatic Diseases*, **8**, 267.

McKUSICK, V. A. (1966), *Hereditable Disorders of Connective Tissue*. St. Louis: Mosby.

MORTON'S METATARSALGIA

An important cause of pain in the foot. Symptoms arise either from a digital neuroma or from pressure of an intermetatarsal bursa on the digital nerve. The latter may be an early manifestation of rheumatoid arthritis. The condition occurs particularly in middle-aged women. It presents with pain in the region of the metatarsal heads which radiates into the toes, relieved by removing the shoe and associated with numbness of the toes. The lesion is most often between the 3rd and 4th metatarsal heads, occasionally the 2nd and 3rd. Examination reveals swelling and tenderness between the metatarsal heads and sometimes diminished sensation over affected toes. A metatarsal pad or injection of the intermetatarsal bursa with prednisolone are sometimes effective. Usually it is necessary to explore the foot and excise the bursa and the digital nerve which is curative.

MSELENI JOINT DISEASE

A degenerative arthropathy found near the Mseleni Mission Hospital in the Ubombo district of northern Zululand. It is believed to represent an unusual type of bone dysplasia, inherited as an autosomal dominant.

Incidence

F. 2 : 1.
Onset in childhood, adolescence, or early adult life.
Affects 25 per cent of men, 66 per cent of women, and about 5 per cent of children in the Mseleni area.

Joints affected

Hips common (80 per cent), knees and ankles in 60 per cent.
Wrists, shoulders, elbows, and hands in 20 per cent.
Bilateral and symmetrical.

Symptoms

Onset of joint pain in childhood, adolescence, or early adult life, usually in hips, knees, or ankles, aggravated by walking.

Signs

Painful limitation of movement; crepitus.
Joints not usually swollen or inflamed.
'Stiff-hipped' gait and lumbar lordosis.

Course

Slowly progressive restriction of movement over many years with increasing pain and eventually inability to walk unaided.

Associations

Slight stunting of growth in some cases.

XR

Changes resemble osteoarthritis: narrowing of joint space, sclerosis of joint margins and osteophytes.
Hip: protrusio acetabuli with deformity and medial subluxation of the femoral head.
In children and adolescents, irregularities and deformities of the epiphyses may be seen.

Laboratory

E.S.R. normal.
Calcium normal.
Phosphates slightly reduced.
Alkaline phosphatase low.

Treatment

As for osteoarthritis: analgesics. Surgery for irreversible changes.

REFERENCES

LOCKITCH, G., and others (1973), *South African Medical Journal*, 47, 2283.

WITTMAN, W., and FELLINGHAM, S A. (1970), *Lancet*, 1, 842.

MUCOPOLYSACCHARIDOSES (MPS)

A group of disorders characterized by accumulation of mucopolysaccharides in tissues. Six types are distinguished, all very rare but Type I commonest; they are inherited as autosomal recessive characters except Type II which is X-linked. Types I, II, III, V, and VI have similar joint manifestations and are considered together. Type IV is considered separately (*see* p. 76). Farber's disease (*see* page 33) is also a mucopolysaccharidosis. (*See also* Winchester Syndrome, p. 150).

Joint manifestations

1. Joint stiffness develops within the first few months of life and leads to claw hands and flexion deformities of other joints within the first few years. All joints are affected; bilateral and symmetrical.
2. Premature osteoarthritis may develop in those who survive into adult life.
3. Carpal tunnel syndrome is a common feature of MPS V.

Associations

MPS I: Hurler syndrome; gargoylism.
1. Dwarfism.
2. Corneal opacity.
3. Mental retardation.
4. Typical coarse 'gargoyle' faces with broad, flattened, saddle nose, large patulous lips, and protruding tongue.
5. Skeletal deformities including kyphosis, short neck, broad hands with short fingers, and genu valgum.
6. Gross hepatosplenomegaly and abdominal herniae.
7. Arterial disease, heart failure, and valve lesions.
Affected children are normal at birth but develop abnormalities within the first year. Death results from respiratory infection or cardiac failure in later childhood.

MPS II: Hunter syndrome.

Similar to MPS I with retinitis pigmentosa, without corneal opacity; milder; males only; survival to about age 40.

MPS III: Sanfilippo syndrome.
1. Mental retardation.
2. Moderate hepatosplenomegaly.
3. Dwarfism but no other skeletal abnormalities.
Survival to about age 40.

MPS V: Scheie syndrome.
1. Corneal opacity with retinitis pigmentosa.
2. Characteristic facies.
3. Aortic valve disease.
Normal stature, intellect, and survival.

MPS VI: Maroteaux-Lamy syndrome.
1. Dwarfism.
2. Hepatosplenomegaly.
3. Anterior sternal protrusion and other skeletal deformities as in MPS I.
4. Corneal opacities.
5. Aortic valve disease.

XR

Developmental abnormalities particularly in skull, vertebrae (wedge-shaped with beaks), ribs, and hands are seen in MPS I, II, and VI.

Laboratory

Increased urinary chondroitin sulphate B (MPS V and VI), heparitin sulphate (MPS III), or both (MPS I and II).
Metachromatic granules often demonstrable in circulating or bone-marrow leucocytes.

Treatment
Symptomatic.

REFERENCE

McKusick, V. A. (1966), *Hereditable Disorders of Connective Tissue*. St. Louis: Mosby.

MULTICENTRIC RETICULOHISTIOCYTOSIS (Lipoid Dermato-arthritis)

A rare condition characterized by a destructive polyarthritis and nodular skin lesions. The diagnosis is made by histological examination of skin or synovium which shows infiltration with giant cells. These cells have a granular 'foamy' cytoplasm containing 'lipoid' material.

Incidence
F. 3 : 1.
Onset in adult life; any age.
Arthritis often precedes skin lesions by a few months or years. Occasionally skin lesions appear first or skin and joint manifestations are synchronous.

Joints affected
Polyarthritis resembling rheumatoid arthritis; affects small joints of hands including D.I.P. joints and knees commonly; often shoulders, wrists, hips, ankles, elbows, feet, and spine; rarely temporomandibular joint.
Bilateral and symmetrical.

Symptoms
Insidious onset of joint pain and swelling.
Bouts of fever, weight-loss.

Signs
Swelling and tenderness.
Later arthritis mutilans of hands with *main-en-lorgnette* and severe deformities resembling those of rheumatoid arthritis.

Course
Chronic with remissions and relapses. Most cases progress at a variable rate to destruction of joints and severe disability often results within a few years.

Associations
1. Chronic skin lesions; yellow, brown, or purple papules or nodules, up to 2 cm. in diameter, particularly situated on dorsum of hands and fingers especially around the nails, forearms, face, ears, and neck. Leonine facies may result. Mucosal nodules in 50 per cent.
2. Xanthelasma palpebrarum (40 per cent).
3. Tendon sheath swellings (20 per cent).

XR
Well-defined translucent areas of bone destruction around affected joints, resembling rheumatoid erosions or cysts. Note involvement of D.I.P. joints. Rarely atlantoaxial subluxation.

Laboratory
E.S.R. may be slightly raised.
Biopsy of skin or synovium confirms.

Treatment
1. Analgesics.
2. Maintain mobility as far as possible.

REFERENCE

BARROW, M. V., and HOLUBAR, K. (1969), *Medicine, Baltimore*, **48**, 287.

MUMPS

A common virus infection, endemic with epidemics every few years, in which an incubation period of 18–21 days is followed by enlargement and tenderness of the parotid glands. The disease occurs predominantly in childhood and though death is exceptional, mumps may be complicated by orchitis, carditis, pancreatitis, meningitis, and encephalitis.

Incidence
M. 7 : 1.
Commoner in adults.
0·5 per cent develop arthritis.
Occasionally a few days before, but usually up to 4 weeks after development of parotitis.

Joints affected
Knees and ankles commonest.
Shoulders, elbows, wrists, M.C.P., and P.I.P. joints often affected.
Occasionally hips and feet.
One or many joints.
Usually asymmetrical. Often migratory.

Symptoms
Pain and swelling; acute onset.

Signs
Variable degree of effusion, erythema, tenderness, and warmth.

Course
Lasts up to 6 weeks.
Complete remission; no sequelae.

Associations
1. Fever.
2. Other complications of mumps, particularly orchitis.

XR
Normal.

Laboratory
Raised E.S.R.
Leucocytosis.
Mumps-complement fixation test positive.
Synovial fluid: inflammatory; polymorph leucocytosis.

Treatment
1. Analgesic and anti-inflammatory drugs. Try indomethacin.
2. ACTH useful if this fails.

REFERENCES

APPELBAUM, E., and others (1952), *Archives of Internal Medicine*, **90**, 217.

LASS, R., and SHEPHARD, E. (1961), *British Medical Journal*, **2**, 1613.

MYCOPLASMA ARTHRITIS

Mycoplasma pneumoniae causes pneumonia which may be accompanied by cold agglutinin haemolytic anaemia. Arthritis is a rare complication. It affects the knees commonly and sometimes ankles, shoulders, and hands, unilateral or bilateral and sometimes migratory. The joints may be normal on examination or a small effusion may be present. The diagnosis is made by finding consolidation on chest X-ray (often extensive despite minimal or absent symptoms and signs), cold agglutinins and a rising complement fixation titre to *M. pneumoniae*. Treatment with tetracycline is followed by complete recovery within a few days without residua.

REFERENCE

LAMBERT, H. P. (1968), *British Medical Journal*, 3, 156.

MYELOMA

Malignant plasma-cell proliferation, characterized by the development of multiple bone tumours. Arthritis is of three types:

1. Due to the presence of myeloma deposits in bone adjacent to joints (*see below*).[1]
2. Associated with amyloidosis (*see p. 5*).
3. Arthritis resembling carcinoma polyarthritis (*see p. 16*).[2]

Incidence

M. = F.
Peak age 50–70.
Bone pain occurs in 90 per cent of cases; pain is localized to joints in 15 per cent.

Joints affected

One or two joints.
Hip commonest.
Occasionally shoulder or knee.
Rarely other large joints.
Unilateral or bilateral.

Symptoms

Persistent pain, often severe, deep and 'boring', often worst at night.

Signs

Painful limitation of movement.
Bone tenderness.

Course

Chronic; usually fatal within a few years.

Associations

1. Bone pain (common), usually in the lumbar or dorsal spine. May cause paraplegia.
2. Infections, particularly pneumonia.
3. Renal failure.

XR

1. Osteolytic deposits adjacent to joints, or in skull or pelvis.
2. Spine: porosis, lytic lesions, collapsed vertebrae.
3. Pathological fractures.

Laboratory

E.S.R. usually over 50 mm. per hour.
Paraprotein on electrophoresis in 75 per cent; diminished levels of immunoglobulins.
Bence Jones proteinuria in 40 per cent.
Bone-marrow: plasma-cell proliferation confirms the diagnosis.
Hypercalcaemia in 50 per cent; alkaline phosphatase usually normal.

Treatment

1. Radiotherapy to painful areas relieves pain.
2. Consider use of melphalan.
3. Analgesics as required; start with simple analgesics and anti-inflammatory drugs; narcotics often necessary later.

REFERENCES

[1] HAMILTON, E. B. D., and BYWATERS, E. G. L. (1961), *Annals of the Rheumatic Diseases*, 20, 353.

[2] DAWSON, A. A. (1966), *Annals of Physical Medicine*, 8, 184.

MYOSITIS OSSIFICANS

A rare condition, inherited as an autosomal dominant of low penetrance, characterized by soft-tissue calcification, eventually leading to complete immobility and death. The condition starts in childhood, usually presenting with localized painful swellings, often accompanied by fever and arthralgia. Diagnosis is made by the radiological finding of sheets of calcification in soft tissues. Congenital skeletal abnormalities, particularly a short big toe or thumb, are commonly found. Treatment with a diphosphonate (disodium etidronate) has been found to prevent progression.

REFERENCES

FLETCHER, E. and MOSS, M. S. (1965), *Annals of the Rheumatic Diseases*, **24**, 267.

RUSSELL, R. G. G., and others (1972), *Lancet*, **1**, 10.

THE NAIL PATELLA SYNDROME

This curious condition affects both mesodermal and ectodermal structures. The principal abnormalities are: (1) Nail changes, the finger nails being one-third or half the normal size, never reaching the finger tips. In some cases the thumb nail is absent or only represented by a fringe of hard keratin in the nail fold, or only the ulnar half is present. In every case the thumb nails are most affected. (2) The patellae are reduced in size or absent. (3) Elbow changes—the carrying angle being increased with limitation of supination and extension. (4) Iliac horns, occasionally palpable. (5) In a minority of cases renal changes with persistent proteinuria, casts of all types and in some cases diminished renal function. The only serious feature is the last, electron microscopy showing changes in the glomerular basement membrane. XR show small or absent patellae, changes in the elbows, a poorly formed subluxated head of the radius articulating with a small underdeveloped capitellum, and iliac bony horns projecting posterolaterally from the centre of the external aspect of the ilium. The bony changes, in fact, cause little inconvenience. The condition is inherited as an autosomal dominant.

REFERENCE

SAMMAN, P. D. (1972), *The Nails in Disease*, 2nd. ed. London: William Heinemann.

NEURALGIC AMYOTROPHY

A condition characterized by pain in the shoulder which may be mistaken for shoulder–hand syndrome (*see* p. 111) or frozen shoulder (*see* p. 34). It is commoner in men (2 : 1) and affects adults with a peak incidence between ages 30 and 50. In about 50 per cent of cases there is some preceding illness, operation, or injury. There is a sudden onset of pain in the shoulder, often very severe; the pain may rarely affect also the elbow and is usually unilateral. Examination at this stage reveals painful limitation of shoulder movement. The pain usually lasts for 1–3 weeks, occasionally up to 3 months, and is followed by evidence of a nerve palsy; the commonest affected nerve is the long thoracic nerve but other upper limb peripheral nerves or nerve-roots may be affected, sometimes with multiple lesions. The neurological lesion recovers slowly over 12–18 months and rarely recurs. Treatment: Analgesics in the acute stage; later physiotherapy to maintain full shoulder movement and restore muscle power in the denervated muscles.

REFERENCE

ALDREN TURNER, J. W., and PARSONAGE, M. J. (1957), *Lancet*, **2**, 209.

NEUROPATHIC JOINT (Charcot's Joint)

Disorganization of a joint and destruction of joint surfaces associated with diminished pain sensation which is most commonly due to: (1) *Tabes dorsalis,* (2) *Diabetes mellitus,* or (3) *Syringomyelia.* Rarely (4) *Hereditary sensory radicular neuropathy and Charcot-Marie-Tooth disease,* (5) *Congenital indifference to pain,* (6) *Spinal cord and peripheral nerve lesions* (traumatic, meningomyelocele, hemiplegia or paraplegia, subacute combined degeneration, leprosy, and yaws), (7) *Familial dysautonomia*[5] (Riley-Day syndrome), (8) *Ulcero-osteolytic neuropathy* in the Bantu.[6]

Incidence

M. 3 : 2.
Usually age 35–65 but also children with congenital lesions.

Joints affected

Depends on localization of pain loss (*see* p. 76).
Affects one to three joints. Monarticular in 70 per cent; asymmetrical in 85 per cent.

Symptoms

50 per cent have acute onset of pain and swelling. 50 per cent insidious swelling and instability.
Pain often absent in the later stages and always less than objective changes would suggest.
May be symptomless.

Signs

Acute stage: warm, red, tender, swollen joint (effusion common).
Chronic stage:
1. Bony swelling and recurrent effusion.
2. Instability—abnormal movements are completely or relatively pain-free.
3. Crepitus on movement.
4. Grotesque deformities eventually develop; sometimes flail joint or marked limb shortening.

Course

Acute inflammatory stage lasts for up to 6 months.

Subsequent slow progression over the years to deformities; disability often minimal despite deformities.
Inflammatory episodes with effusion occur occasionally during course of disease.
Complications:
1. Infection.
2. Fracture.
3. Haemorrhage.
4. Local nerve or cord compression.
5. Dislocation.

XR

1. Sclerosis of bone ends.
2. Realinement and remodelling, which may result in bizarre shapes of bone ends.
3. Loss of joint space.
4. Loose bodies.
5. Massive osteophytes.
6. Periarticular calcification.
7. Fractures.

Laboratory

E.S.R. normal.
Synovial fluid: non-inflammatory.

Treatment

1. Rest in acute stage.
2. Avoid trauma.
3. Stabilization by braces, callipers, and splints to prevent or correct deformity.
4. Consider arthrodesis for intractable pain, gross instability, or pressure on nerves, but bony union may fail to occur.

CONDITIONS ASSOCIATED WITH NEUROPATHIC JOINTS

TABES DORSALIS[2]

Incidence

5 per cent have neuropathic joint.

Joints affected

Lower limb (98 per cent).
Knee commonest (70 per cent).
Ankle, hip, and feet (30 per cent).
Vertebral (20 per cent)—lumbar or lower thoracic.
Rarely elbow or shoulder (2 per cent).

Associations

Argyll Robertson pupil in 80 per cent.
Absent knee- and ankle-jerks, loss of pain sensation and joint position sense, ataxia.

Laboratory

W.R. (20 per cent negative in blood and C.S.F.) and T.P.I.

SYRINGOMYELIA[3]

Incidence

25 per cent have neuropathic joint.

Joints affected

Upper limb (80 per cent).
Shoulder commonest (30 per cent).
Elbow (25 per cent); wrist or thumb (20 per cent).
Ankle or knee (15 per cent).
Rarely hip, temporomandibular or sterno-clavicular joint.
50 per cent have cervical spondylosis on X-ray.

Associations

Loss of pain and temperature sensation (other modalities intact) in upper limbs, upper trunk, and 'Balaclava helmet' distribution.
Wasting of small muscles of hands.
Spastic paraparesis.

Laboratory

Unhelpful.
C.S.F. normal.

DIABETES MELLITUS[4]

Incidence

0·1 per cent of all diabetics and 5 per cent of those with diabetic neuropathy have neuropathic joint.

Joints affected

Foot in 80 per cent; tarsal and M.T.P. joints commonest.
Occasionally ankle (10 per cent).
Rarely knee or lumbar vertebrae.

Associations

Long-standing diabetes.
Sensory loss (all modalities) in glove and stocking distribution.
Absent ankle-jerks.
Retinopathy common.
Trophic ulceration and soft tissue or bone infection.

Laboratory

Hyperglycaemia; glycosuria.

REFERENCES

[1] STOREY, G. O. (1970), *Rheumatology and Physical Medicine*, **10**, 312.

[2] STEINDLER, A., and others (1942), *The Urologic and Cutaneous Review*, **46**, 633.

[3] SCHLESINGER, H. (1895), *Die Syringomyelie*. Leipzig and Vienna: Deuticke.

[4] ROBILLARD, R., and others (1964), *Canadian Medical Association Journal*, **91**, 795.

[5] BRUNT, P. W. (1967), *British Medical Journal*, **4**, 277.

[6] ANDERSON, I. F., and SCHULZ, E. J. (1971), *British Journal of Dermatology*, **85**, Supplement 7, 18.

NON-DISEASE

Occurs in rheumatology as in other disciplines. Examples are aches and pains associated with degenerative changes in the cervical spine on XR (non-cervical spondylitis), hyperuricaemia (non-gout), false-positive latex test (non-rheumatoid arthritis), or weakly positive A.N.F. (non-S.L.E.). The importance of non-disease lies in its potential conversion to real disease by the exhibition of toxic and unnecessary drugs.

REFERENCE

MEADOR, C. K. (1965), *New England Journal of Medicine*, **272**, 92.

OCCUPATIONAL ARTHROPATHIES

There are many ways in which patients' occupations may lead to joint disease.[1] They include:

1. *Osteoarthritis.* Though trauma and 'wear and tear' may not be the basic cause of osteoarthritis, it is certainly one factor and may influence the site of the disease. Thus cotton workers have a higher incidence of osteoarthritis of the hands and neck, while coal workers have it in the knees and lumbar spine.[2] The following is a selection of sites of osteoarthritis related to repeated occupational trauma:

Wicket-keeper's hand, affecting all small joints but especially the distal interphalangeals. Baseball-catcher's hand. Goalkeeper's fingers, related to repeated hyperextension of the fingers to deflect the ball over the crossbar. Bricklayer's hands. Family-planner's fingers—middle and index on the right hand. Seamstresses fingers.

Cello or bass player's thumb, affecting the first carpometacarpal joint. Ticket clipper's thumb in railway inspectors.

Driller's wrist. Yoga wrist.

Puppeteer's elbow.

Chauffeur's shoulder.

Porter's neck:[3] injuries sustained while carrying heavy loads on the head may lead to pain and stiffness but also to spinal cord compression.

Labourer's spine.

Zulu dancer's hip.

Fast-bowler's foot, affecting the ankle and mid-tarsus.

Nurse's foot. Ballet-dancer's foot.

2. *Traumatic tenosynovitis or peritendonitis* occurs particularly in occupations requiring repetition of stereotyped movements. It occurs particularly after a period away from work or in newcomers, for example in the forearm, wrist or fingers of hop-pickers (hopper's gout) or haymakers. There is pain, limitation of movement, tense localized swelling, tenderness and sometimes warmth and erythema. Crepitus is felt over the affected tendon during movement. The condition lasts for a few days or weeks but it may recur when the patient resumes his occupation. Treatment: (1) Rest; (2) Local injection of prednisolone.

3. *Occupational bursitis:* pressure, friction or repeated trauma causes swelling, usually chronic and painless but occasionally with acute painful episodes which may be due to superimposed infection. There are numerous bursae, 156 in the body[4,5] and the condition can occur in any of them. The following varieties have achieved names:

Olecranon bursitis: miner's elbow, beat elbow, student's elbow, drunkard's (boozer's) elbow.

Ischial bursitis: weaver's bottom.

Prepatellar bursitis: housemaid's knee, nun's knee, beat knee, carpet-layer's knee.

Subachromial bursitis: hod-carrier's shoulder. Adventitious bursae may form and the same problem arises, for example over the vertex (Covent Garden hummy), over the 7th cervical spine (humper's lump, Billingsgate hump), over the upper part of the shoulder (dustman's shoulder) or over the external malleolus (tailor's ankle).

4. *Carpal tunnel syndrome* (p. 22) is particularly common in those whose occupations involve repeated movements such as operating a machine.

5. So called *tennis elbow, golfer's elbow* and other enthesopathies are commonly precipitated by repetitive movements at work.

6. *Poisoning*. Brassfounder's ague (metal fume fever, Monday fever) and polymer fume fever are acute reactions to inhalation of particles in which arthralgia may be a prominent feature There is fever with rigors, sweating, and headache. Attacks last about 48 hours and may recur with repeated exposure.
   Vinyl chloride poisoning causes acro-osteolysis (p. 2) with Raynaud's phenomenon and skin changes resembling scleroderma.[6] Pains in joints and muscles may occur in acute lead poisoning. Chronic lead poisoning causes secondary (saturnine) gout.

7. *Infections*. Fish-filleter's fingers are due to infection with *Erysipelothrix rhusiopathiae* (erysipeloid). There is local pain and swelling but the condition is usually mild. It resolves spontaneously within a few weeks and responds to penicillin. See also sporotrichosis (p. 35). Beat hand is a cellulitis occuring in miners and stokers.
   See also Avascular necrosis in divers and caisson workers (p. 10); Gamekeeper's thumb (p. 36).

REFERENCES

[1] HUNTER, D. (1962), *The Diseases of Occupations*. London: English Universities Press.
[2] KELLGREN, J. H., and LAWRENCE, J. S. (1958), *Annals of the Rheumatic Diseases*, 17, 388.
[3] LEVY, L. L. (1968), *British Medical Journal*, 2, 16.
[4] MONRO, A. SECUNDUS (1788), 'a Description of all the Bursae Mucosae of the Human Body', Edinburgh: Eliot.
[5] BYWATERS, E. G. L. (1965), 'The Bursae of the Body', *Annals of the Rheumatic Diseases*, 24, 215.
[6] WALKER, A. (1975), *Proceedings of the Royal Society of Medicine*, 68, 343.

OCHRONOSIS

A rare hereditary disease in which deficiency of the enzyme homogentisic acid oxidase is transmitted as an autosomal recessive character. The condition was described independently as *alkaptonuria* because of the excretion in urine of 'alkaptan', later identified as homogentisic acid, and as *ochronosis* because of the accumulation of pigment in tissues. Spondylitis and a degenerative arthropathy are features of the disease, probably caused by the presence of pigment in cartilage.

Incidence

M. 2 : 1; males affected more severely.
Onset usually at age 20–40 in men, 40–50 in women.
F.H. common. Inquire for consanguinity.

Joints affected

Spine usually.
Knees commonly (80 per cent).
Often shoulders (50 per cent) and hips (50 per cent).
Bilateral and symmetrical.

Symptoms

1. Insidious onset of back pain and stiffness.
2. Pain in knees follows 10–20 years later with other peripheral joints 10 years later still; stiffness; limitation of movement.

Signs

Spine: Tenderness over lumbar vertebrae, loss of lumbar lordosis, thoracic kyphosis. Later limitation of movement and chest expansion—note resemblance to ankylosing spondylitis.
Joints: Bony swelling of knees with later development of restriction of movement, crepitus, and flexion contracture. Intermittent effusion.

Course

Chronic, usually progressing to disablement (due to spinal and knee involvement) in about 20 years.
Acute episodes occur following minor trauma to peripheral joints or because of vertebral disc herniation which occurs in 20 per cent of men at some time.

OCHRONOSIS (*continued*)

Associations
1. Black, dark-brown, or bluish discoloration of ear cartilages (sometimes also tinnitus or deafness), sclerae, cornea, conjunctiva, eyelids, and skin (particularly sweat-producing areas). Usually appears at age 30–40, but rarely as early as childhood.
2. Renal and prostatic calculi.
3. Urine which becomes black on standing (or when alkalinized).

XR
Spine: Calcification of intervertebral discs; later narrowing of disc spaces with sclerosis of adjacent vertebral margins; still later discs disappear and vertebrae fuse.
Sacro-iliac joints: Normal.
No ligamentous calcification.
Peripheral joints: Narrowing of joint space, irregular joint surface with sclerosis, cystic changes, and osteophytes.
Occasionally loose bodies and calcification of soft tissues (hydroxyapatite).

Laboratory
Confirm presence of homogentisic acid in urine.

Treatment
Analgesics.

REFERENCE

O'BRIEN, W. M., and others (1963), *American Journal of Medicine*, 34, 813.

ONCHOCERCIASIS

Onchocerca volvulus infection, found on the coasts of West and East Africa and in parts of South America. Microfilariae are introduced into the skin by the bite of a female black fly (buffalo gnat), and form a granulomatous nodule. Migration of microfilariae into the eye causes inflammatory lesions (keratitis, corneal opacity, iritis, choroidoretinitis) and may lead to blindness. Arthritis is due to migration of microfilariae into the joint and resembles septic arthritis.

Incidence
M. = F.
Adults.
Arthritis is rare.

Joints affected
Knee or hip.
Monarticular.

Symptoms
Sudden onset of severe pain and swelling as in septic arthritis, but patient feels well.

Signs
Affected joint is red, warm, tender, and swollen with effusion.
Pain on movement but limitation less striking than with septic arthritis.
Fever usual.

Course
Arthritis lasts up to 2 weeks, and recovers completely without residua.

Associations
1. Skin nodules of onchocerciasis always present, but not necessarily near the joint.
2. Sometimes eye lesions.

XR
Normal.

Laboratory
Synovial fluid: W.B.C. raised, predominantly neutrophils.
Microscopy shows microfilariae.
Fluid should be examined immediately after aspiration.

Treatment
1. Analgesics.
2. Aspiration of fluid, repeated if necessary.
3. Diethylcarbamazine or suramin; low initial dose if eyes are involved.
4. Removal of skin lesions if troublesome.

REFERENCE

DEJOU, L. (1939), *Presse médicale*, 47, 983.

OSGOOD-SCHLATTER'S DISEASE

A condition resembling tennis elbow but occurring at the attachment of the patellar tendon to the tibial tubercle. It occurs particularly in boys (8 : 1) at age 10–15 and especially those with unusual sporting prowess. There is pain in the tibial tubercle aggravated by exercise. Examination reveals a tender enlarged tibial tubercle. The condition lasts for up to one year and resolves spontaneously. Recurrence is rare. Treatment: Explanation of the nature of the condition, reassurance of the absence of arthritis, rest, simple analgesics and local injection of prednisolone.

OSTEITIS PUBIS

A non-suppurative inflammation of the symphysis pubis which is a rare sequel to pelvic surgery or childbirth, particularly when these are complicated by infection. It has been reported particularly after prostatectomy, gynaecological operations, and bladder surgery, but also rarely after childbirth, herniorrhaphy, rectal surgery, prostatic abscess, pyelonephritis, and abortion. The condition must be distinguished from osteomyelitis and from ankylosing spondylitis.

Incidence

M. = F.
Peak age 40–60.
Onset usually 2–30 days after operation; rarely up to $1\frac{1}{2}$ years.

Joints affected

Pubic symphysis.

Symptoms

Burning or boring pain in the anterior pelvic area; sometimes also felt in ischial tuberosities, groins, perineum, and adductor region of thighs.
Aggravated by walking, sneezing, coughing, and sitting.

Signs

1. Painful restriction of hip movement.
2. Tenderness over the symphysis pubis.
3. Waddling gait. Walking backwards may be preferable to walking forwards. Patient prefers to remain in bed with hips flexed.

Course

Persists for weeks or months untreated.
Usually responds well to treatment.

Associations

Urinary infection in 30 per cent.

XR

Normal for the first few weeks.
Symphysis pubis shows local porosis and erosions, producing a 'moth-eaten' appearance. Later there is sclerosis of the joint margins.
Sacro-iliac joints normal.

Laboratory

W.B.C. and E.S.R. usually slightly raised.
Urinary infection in 30 per cent.

Treatment

1. Anti-inflammatory drugs: phenylbutazone indomethacin, or occasionally steroids.
2. Antibiotics for urinary or wound infection.
3. Surgical drainage required for osteo-myelitis or retropubic abscess formation.
4. Arthrodesis or wedge resection of the symphysis if all else fails.

REFERENCES

BARNES, W. C., and MALAMENT, M. (1963), *Surgery, Gynecology and Obstetrics*, **117**, 277.

COVENTRY, M. B., and MITCHELL, W. C. (1961), *Journal of the American Medical Association*, **178**, 898.

OSTEOARTHRITIS (Osteoarthrosis)

A disorder of cartilage with characteristic histological, clinical and radiological features. The histological changes include flaking of the surface of cartilage (fibrillation), the appearance of vertical fissures and proliferation of chondrocytes which form nests around the fissures. Electron microscopy shows the presence of increased numbers of matrix vesicles which are the site of formation of crystals of hydroxyapatite. There is progressive loss of cartilage and secondary changes in subchondral bone, fibrosis of the capsule, and mild inflammatory changes in synovium. Various biochemical changes suggest that the disease may be a metabolic abnormality of cartilage. There is increased water content, loss of proteoglycans, increased levels of potentially destructive enzymes like cathepsin D and increased excretion of alkaline phosphatase and pyrophosphatase. Some condition appear to lead to osteoarthritis or to determine its occurrence at a particular site (secondary osteoarthritis):

1. *Congenital anatomical aberrations of joints:* Hypermobility. Abnormally shaped or positioned surfaces.

2. *Structural disorders arising in children:* Perthes' disease (p. 96). Slipped femoral epiphysis.

3. *Trauma and mechanical problems:* Fractures involving the joint surface. Meniscectomy. Obesity. Recurrent dislocation. Occupational hazards (p. 85).

4. *Crystal deposition disease:* Pyrophosphate arthropathy. Gout.

5. *Metabolic abnormalities of cartilage:* Ochronosis (p. 86).

6. *Avascular necrosis.*

7. *Other conditions in which cartilage is destroyed* including septic arthritis and recurrent haemarthrosis in haemophilia.

In most cases, the disease is primary, without obvious predisposing cause:

Incidence
VERY COMMON—about 20 per cent have it.
F.2:1.
Peak onset age 50, usually 40–65.
50 per cent of the population have XR changes—almost universal after age 55.
About 50 per cent of patients with XR changes have symptoms.
F.H. in 40 per cent.
Inheritance probably multifactorial.

Joints involved
Knees (75 per cent) and hands (60 per cent) commonest.
In the hands, DIP joints and carpo-metacarpal joints of thumbs are commonest with P.I.P. joints (50 per cent) less prominent and M.C.P. joints unusual. Feet in 40 per cent, usually 1st M.T.P. joint—other M.T.P. joints less commonly.
Lumbar (30 per cent) and cervical spine (20 per cent) often—hips (25 per cent), ankles (20 per cent), shoulders (15 per cent)—rarely elbows or wrists. 10 per cent monarticular.
Usually 1,2,3, or 4 sites. Bilateral in 85 per cent—when one is affected first or more severely, it is usually the dominant side.

Symptoms
Pain, worst towards evening and aggravated by particular activities. 80 per cent have morning stiffness (usually 10–30 min. and seldom more than 60 min.—localized to one or two sites) and inactivity stiffness (usually 5 min. and seldom more than 30 min.).

Signs
Knee: Bony swelling, effusions in 60 per cent, Baker's cyst (40 per cent), tenderness, painful limitation of movement, crepitus.
D.I.P. Joints: Joints often red, warm and exquisitely tender in acute stage ('hot Heberden's nodes'). After months or years inflammatory features pass leaving bony swelling and sometimes flexion, valgus or varus deformities.
C.M.C. Joint: 'Square hand' with bony swelling, tenderness and crepitus of joint.
Others: Bony swelling, tenderness, crepitus, painful limitation of movement.

Course:
Chronic additive pattern. Slowly progressive with exacerbations and remissions. Affected joints develop progressive painful restriction of movement, sometimes with deformities (hip—flexion; knee—valgus) or laxity. Greatest disability in late stages results from involvement of weight-bearing joints.

Associations
No extra-articular features.

XR
1. Loss of joint space.
2. Sclerosis of adjacent bone.
3. Marginal osteophytes.
4. Subarticular cysts.

5. 'Spotty' calcification indicates hydroxy-apatite deposition. Seen in the hands in 60 per cent, usually D.I.P. joints, and knees in 25 per cent. 'Linear' calcification (chondrocalcinosis) indicates pyrophosphate deposition (*see* p. 108).

Warning: These changes are universal after age 55 and are therefore found in patients with serious conditions like polymyalgia and malignancy.

Laboratory

E.S.R. normal.

Latex negative (but 5 per cent positive in normal elderly people).

No diagnostic tests.

Synovial fluid: clear and viscous ('non-inflammatory'). Usually about 3000 (up to 15,000) $\times 10^9$ cells/dl. Typically 80 per cent mononuclear (40–100 per cent). Look for pyrophosphate crystals under polarised light. Electron microscopy may show crystals of hydroxyapatite.

Treatment

1. Analgesic and anti-inflammatory drugs to relieve pain. Start with propionic acid derivatives. Simple analgesics on demand for patients with mild or intermittent pain.
2. Surgery in severe cases.
   Hip: Total replacement.
   Knee: Replacement or osteotomy to relieve pain and correct deformity.
   C.M.C. Joint: Trapezectomy or fusion.
3. Physical measures. Walking stick. Reduce weight by dieting. Physiotherapy to maintain muscle power and range of movement. Hydrotherapy for painful stiff hips.

REFERENCES

EHRLICH, G. E., and others (1975), *Journal of the American Medical Association*, **232**, 157.

HOWELL, D. S., and others (1976), *Seminars in Arthritis and Rheumatism*, **5**, 365.

KELLGREN, J. H., and MOORE, R. (1952), *British Medical Journal*, **1**, 181.

LAURENCE, J. S., and others (1966), *Annals of Rheumatic Diseases*, **25**, 1.

OSTEOCHONDRITIS DISSECANS

A condition characterized by the separation of avascular osteochondral fragments from the surface of joints. If separation is complete, loose bodies are found within the joint. The condition is thought to result from traumatic fractures of the joint surface.

Incidence

M. 2 : 1.
Peak age 10–20 (5–60).
Common in sportsmen: sometimes familial.

Joints affected

Knee commonest (85 per cent).
Elbow or ankle (10 per cent).
Rarely M.T.P. joint or hip.
Unilateral in 75 per cent. Usually only one site.

Symptoms

1. Pain, often mild, worse after exercise.
2. Recurrent swelling.
3. Feeling of instability and 'giving way'.
4. 'Locking'.
History of preceding injury in 40 per cent.

Signs

Often none.
Effusion occasionally with muscle wasting and slight joint tenderness.
Occasionally there are mechanical abnormalities (valgus, varus, recurvatum), instability or dislocation of patella.

Course

Acute episode recovers within a few months. Osteoarthritis follows after a few years in 50 per cent.

XR

1. Separation of a fragment or fragments of bone from joint surface.
2. Sclerosis of the fragment and of the crater from which it came.
3. Rarely osteochondral fracture.
4. Osteoarthritic changes later.
Commonest site is lateral border of medial femoral condyle.

Laboratory

Unhelpful.

Treatment

1. Immobilization in a non-weight-bearing plaster for mild cases. Spontaneous healing more likely in younger cases. Assess by regular X-ray.
2. Surgery. *Early*: fixation of the fragment before complete separation has occurred. *Late*: removal of loose bodies.

REFERENCE

AICROTH, P. (1971), *Journal of Bone and Joint Surgery*, **53B**, 440.

OSTEOCHONDROMATOSIS

A rare condition characterized by the formation of foci of cartilage in the synovial membrane. These become detached to form loose bodies. The cartilage is often calcified and sometimes ossified.

Incidence
M. 2 : 1.
Any age, peak 20–40.

Joints affected
Knee or hip commonest (75 per cent).
Rarely shoulder, ankle, or elbow.
Usually monarticular.

Symptoms
Episodes of pain, stiffness, and sometimes swelling.
'Locking' or 'giving way'.

Signs
Swelling due to effusion and synovial thickening.
Limitation of movement.
Crepitus; loose bodies may be palpable.

Course
Recurrent painful episodes.
May lead to secondary osteoarthritis.

XR
Usually shows multiple small opacities (rarely not seen because they are not calcified), producing a 'stippled effect'.
Loose bodies.
Joint surfaces normal until late when degenerative changes develop.

Laboratory
Histology confirms (synovial biopsy).

Treatment
1. Removal of loose bodies.
2. Synovectomy of the knee.

Loose bodies
Osteochondral loose bodies are also found in osteochondritis dissecans and rarely in osteoarthritis, neuropathic joints, and avascular necrosis.
Fibrinous loose bodies are found in any chronic synovitis such as rheumatoid arthritis.

REFERENCE

JEFFREYS, T. E. (1967), *Journal of Bone and Joint Surgery*, **49B**, 530.

OSTEOMALACIA and RICKETS

Bone lesions adjacent to joints may cause arthritis as in hyperparathyroidism (*see* p. 54). Bone pain may also simulate arthritis; it is felt particularly in the back, groins, and thighs, is aggravated by weight-bearing and relieved by rest, and responds to treatment with vitamin D.

REFERENCE

STANBURY, S. W., and others (1959), *Annals of the Rheumatic Diseases*, **18**, 63.

PAGET'S DISEASE (Osteitis deformans)

A disorder of unknown aetiology affecting one or many bones, particularly the pelvis, femur, skull, tibia and vertebrae. The condition is rare before the age of 30, rising thereafter from 0·5 per cent at 40 years to 10 per cent at 90 years. 5 per cent of patients with radiological changes also have symptoms, usually bone pain and deformities.

Four types of arthritis may occur: (1) Arthritis as a result of disease adjacent to the joint, described *below*. (2) Calcific periarthritis (p. 15). (3) Acute gout (p. 39). (4) Ankylosing spondylitis-like illness with pain, stiffness, limitation of spinal movement but negative HLA B27.

Incidence
M. 2 : 1.
Age 40+.
F. H. often.

Joints affected
Hips, knees, lumbar and dorsal spine.
7 per cent bilateral.

Symptoms
1. Dull, aching pain aggravated by use or immobility.
2. Stiffness after rest in 50 per cent.

Signs
Hip: limitation of movement.
Knees: bony swelling, warmth, limitation of movement and crepitus.

Course
Chronic and slowly progressive; end-result resembles severe osteoarthritis.

Associations
Other features of Paget's disease; large skull, bowed tibia, deafness, kyphosis.
Rarely spinal cord, nerve root or cauda equina compression, high output cardiac failure, and osteogenic sarcoma.

XR
1. *Bone:* first change is localized porosis (in skull, so-called 'osteoporosis circumscripta'). Later there is replacement of normal bone by coarse dense trabeculae. Bone often expanded and thickened.

2. *Hip:* narrowing of joint space; osteophytes occasionally with bony bridging; deepening of acetabulum leading to protrusio acetabuli in 20 per cent.
3. *Knee:* narrowing of joint space, osteophytes.
4. *Spine:* vertebrae show sclerosis or collapse.
5. Fractures of long bones.
6. Periarticular calcification.

Laboratory
Alkaline phosphatase usually elevated (heat labile); calcium usually normal.
Urinary hydroxyproline excretion > 40 mg/24 hr. Hyperuricaemia in 40 per cent, particularly males—about half of these (40 per cent) have episodes of acute gout. Bone biopsy rarely required to confirm the diagnosis and exclude malignant disease.

Treatment
1. Analgesics.
2. Specific therapy with Calcitonin, Mithramycin or EHDP. Calcitonin (Salmon) 100 u. I.M. daily for 3–6 months then maintenace 50 u. three times weekly if it works (or porcine 160 u. daily with maintenance 80 u.). Mithramycin 15 mg./kg.I.V. daily for 10 days. Give it over 6 hours in 5 per cent dextrose. Check calcium and liver function tests daily. Remission should last years. EHDP 20 mg./kg/day by month. Stop after 3 to 6 months and give another course if it recurs.
3. Treatment of complications, e.g., fractures.

REFERENCES

FRANCK, W. A., and others (1974), *American Journal of Medicine*, **56**, 592.
MACHTEY, I., and others (1966), *American Journal of the Medical Sciences*, **251**, 524.

RUSSELL, A. S., and DENTLE, B. C. (1974), *Canadian Medical Association Journal*, **110**, 397.
RUSSELL, R. G. G., and others (1974), *Lancet*, **2**, 894.

PAINFUL FAT KNEES IN SHORT FAT LADIES

It is common for short fat ladies to have painful fat knees. Osteoarthritis is usually present in fat-festooned lower extremities (grand piano legs), which are unsightly, often oedematous, and extremely demoralizing to the sufferer. A tender pad of fat is found over the medial side of the knee but tenderness also occurs elsewhere over fatty and other soft tissues. Therapy including diet, analgesics, and diuretics is usually unrewarding.

REFERENCE

DIXON, A. ST. J. (1965), *Progress in Clinical Rheumatology*. London: Churchill.

PALINDROMIC RHEUMATISM

A condition characterized by recurrent, acute, but self-limiting, attacks of arthritis.[1,2]

Incidence
M. = F.
Age 15 + . Typical onset age 30.

Joints affected
Hands, wrists, knees, and feet commonly.
Shoulders, ankles, and elbows often.
Hips and jaws occasionally.
May affect big toe resembling gout.
Each patient tends to have one to three favourite sites.

Symptoms
Sudden onset of severe pain and stiffness.

Signs
Swollen, red, tender joint.
Periarticular soft tissues may be involved.
No fever.

Course
Attacks occur at irregular intervals, average 20 per year. There may be many years of freedom between attacks or hundreds of attacks in one year.
Attacks last a few hours or days, seldom more than one week.
Complete recovery follows the attack. 50 per cent of patients continue to have episodic arthritis, 35 per cent develop typical rheumatoid arthritis, a few develop S.L.E. or remit.

XR
Normal.

Laboratory
E.S.R. may be raised in acute attack.
Latex test positive in 50 per cent.

Treatment
1. Indomethacin, phenylbutazone, or aspirin for acute attacks.
2. Gold or penicillamine therapy may produce remission. Penicillamine: 250 mg. daily usually sufficient.[3]

REFERENCES

[1]HENCH, P. S., and ROSENBERG, E. F. (1944), *Archives of Internal Medicine*, **73**, 293.
[2]MATTINGLY, S. (1966), *Annals of the Rheumatic Diseases*, **25**, 307.
[3]HUSKISSON, E. C. (1976), *British Medical Journal*, **2**, 979.

ACUTE PANCREATITIS or PANCREATIC CARCINOMA

These diseases are rarely accompanied by tender nodular skin lesions due to subcutaneous fat necrosis, which resemble erythema nodosum, but occur on the thighs and buttocks and occasionally over the upper limbs, trunk, and scalp as well as in the typical skin distribution. This may be associated with a transient polyarthritis.

Incidence

M. 3 : 1.
Age 30–60 with pancreatitis, 50–80 with carcinoma.
Arthritis is synchronous with skin lesions; may precede other manifestations by several weeks.

Joints affected

Ankles (65 per cent), knees (50 per cent), and small joints of hands (50 per cent) commonest.
Occasionally elbows (30 per cent), wrists, toes, and shoulders.
Rarely hips and temporomandibular joints.
Usually polyarticular.
Symmetrical in 65 per cent.

Symptoms

Acute onset of pain and swelling.

Signs

Joints often warm, red, and swollen.

Course

Arthritis resolves completely within a few weeks; no residua. Also relieved by successful surgery.

Associations

1. Nodular skin lesions (*see above*).
2. Alcoholism, gall-stones, or abdominal trauma may predispose to pancreatitis.

XR

Normal.

Laboratory

Raised serum amylase.
Eosinophilia.
Skin biopsy shows fat necrosis.

Treatment

1. Anti-inflammatory drugs.
2. Surgery may be required.

REFERENCE

Mullin, G. T., and others (1968), *Annals of Internal Medicine*, **68**, 75.

PERIOSTITIS DEFORMANS

A rare condition characterized by the formation of multiple periosteal tumours. These appear in the long bones and are usually bilateral and symmetrical. There is a sudden onset of local swelling, sometimes painful, followed by gradual disappearance of the swelling over the next few months. Attacks recur at irregular intervals throughout the patient's lifetime, usually several years apart, and tend to become less severe with time. XR show a localized ossified periosteal proliferation. Large osteophytes develop around joints and deformities may result. Treatment is symptomatic.

REFERENCE

SORIANO, M. (1952), *Annals of the Rheumatic Diseases*, **11**, 154.

PERTHES' DISEASE (Legg-Calvé-Perthes' Disease or Coxa Plana)

Idiopathic avascular necrosis of the epiphysis of the head of the femur, a distinct clinical syndrome causing hip pain in children and important in the differential diagnosis of juvenile arthritis and tuberculosis.

Incidence
M. 5 : 1.
Peak age 6–8; not before 3 or after 16.
6 per cent familial.
Rare in Negroes.

Joints affected
Hip only.
10 per cent bilateral. One hip may follow the other after several years.

Symptoms
Pain in the hip or knee—varies from severe to mild or absent.
Limp.

Signs
Painful limitation of movement.

Course
Acute phase lasts for weeks or months then settles spontaneously. 75 per cent of cases do well with little or no residual disability. A few are left with shortening of the leg, hip deformity or limitation of movement; 20 per cent develop premature osteoarthritis; 10 per cent will eventually require hip replacement.
Prognosis related to age of onset—under 6 always good; not related to initial severity. Development of osteoarthritis related to eventual shape of femoral head.

Associations
None

XR
1. Normal at first. Then:
2. A crescent of radiolucency forms parallel to the surface of the femoral head. The fragment of bone may later separate.
3. Increased density of femoral head.
4. In severe cases there may be areas of radiolucency in the femoral head or fragmentation of the epiphysis.
5. Eventually there is remodelling leaving a flattened femoral head, a short broad femoral neck and an enlarged acetabulum.

Laboratory
No abnormality.

Treatment
No universal agreement.
Possibilities include:
1. None—certainly best in young children who do well anyway.
2. Traction in the acute stage, then 'broomstick plasters' to maintain abduction and internal rotation. Frames and callipers are no longer used.
3. Osteotomy may be considered to achieve the same position as broomstick plasters, avoiding prolonged immobilisation.

REFERENCES

CATTERALL, A. (1971), *Journal of Bone and Joint Surgery*, **53B**, 37.
GOWER, W. E., and JOHNSTONE, R. C. (1971), *Journal of Bone and Joint Surgery*, **53A**, 759.

SOMERVILLE, E. W. (1971), *Journal of Bone and Joint Surgery*, **53B**, 639.

PIGMENTED VILLONODULAR SYNOVITIS

A rare, non-malignant condition characterized by synovial proliferation, pigmentation with haemosiderin, the formation of grape-like nodular masses, villi, and pannus. The diagnosis should be considered in a patient with chronic synovitis of one joint.

Incidence
M.=F.
Any age, particularly young adults.

Joints affected
Knee commonest.
Occasionally foot, ankle, or finger.
Rarely hip, elbow, wrist, or shoulder.
Usually monarticular.

Symptoms
Insidious onset of joint swelling over several years.
Pain is usually mild or absent.
There may be attacks of joint pain, sometimes related to trauma.

Signs
1. Swelling due to synovial thickening.
2. In acute episodes the joint may be warm and tender with effusion.
3. Limitation of movement.
4. Occasionally there are localized swellings around the joints, related to tendons.

Course
Chronic with acute exacerbations which recur at irregular intervals, months or years apart.
Severe disability may result after many years.

Associations
No systemic manifestations.

XR
Usually normal.
Degenerative changes may be seen and rarely areas of porosis adjacent to the joint, resembling malignant deposits, or joint surface erosions.

Laboratory
Raised E.S.R. in exacerbations.
Synovial fluid: blood-stained and xanthochromic.
Synovial biopsy: nodular proliferation, haemosiderosis, infiltration with mononuclear cells.
Latex test negative.

Treatment
Synovectomy alleviates; about 30 per cent recur and the operation should only be advised if symptoms are troublesome.

Variants
Nodular type: nodular lesions occur usually on the fingers, not causing arthritis; excision is curative.

REFERENCE

BYERS, P. D., and others (1968), *Journal of Bone and Joint Surgery*, **50B**, 290.

PLANT THORN SYNOVITIS

An inflammatory arthritis caused by the presence within a joint of plant thorns. It is important since it may be confused with juvenile chronic arthritis but is completely curable by synovectomy. Typically a child kneels on a thorn, may not even notice it, but later develops arthritis of that particular joint.

Incidence
Rare.
Usually children aged 4–7.
Arthritis starts up to 3 weeks after the injury.
Commonest in late summer and autumn.

Joints affected
Usually one knee.
Monarticular.

Symptoms
Pain, swelling and stiffness.

Signs
Affected joint is swollen and warm with effusion and synovial thickening. Sometimes fever.

Course
Chronic but resolves completely after synovectomy.

Associations
None.

XR
Usually normal.
Radiolucent 'pseudocysts' of bone adjacent to the joint described.

Laboratory
Raised E.S.R.
Synovial fluid: inflammatory W.B.C. up to $30,000 \times 10^9$/dl., mostly polymorphs. May grow irrelevant organisms (secondary infection). Synovial biopsy: synovial hypertrophy; infiltration with lymphocytes and plasma cells; granulomatous lesions with foreign body giant cells containing vegetable material which is identified by polarized light or PAS stain.

Treatment
Complete synovectomy.
Antibiotics, anti-inflammatory drugs and intra-articular corticosteroids are ineffective.

REFERENCE

SUGERMAN, M., and others (1977), *Arthritis and Rheumatism*, **20**, 1125.

POLIOMYELITIS

An epidemic virus infection with an incubation period of 2–3 weeks. There is a mild, prodromal illness with malaise and fever lasting for a few days and followed by lymphocytic meningitis, pain in the limbs, and, in some cases, paralysis. The disease has become rarer and milder in recent years.

Incidence
M. = F.
Children and young adults affected.
Arthritis is rare.
Arthritis commonly appears with the onset of paralysis but rarely up to a few weeks later.

Joints affected
Typically one joint in a paralysed limb— sometimes polyarticular.
Knees and ankles commonest.
Occasionally hips, elbows, wrists, M.C.P. or interphalangeal joints.
Usually only joints of paralysed limbs.

Symptoms
Pain, often severe.
Swelling.

Signs
Swelling and diffuse tenderness of joint and muscles.
Joints sometimes warm but not red.

Course
Joint remains swollen for weeks or months, but usually resolves completely.
Ankylosis is a rare sequel.

Associations
Paralysis of limbs with flaccidity, and loss of reflexes, developing over a few days with no loss of sensation.

XR
Early: normal.
Later: porosis; rarely diminution of joint space or ankylosis.

Laboratory
C.S.F.: early polymorph leucocytosis.
Later lymphocytosis. Slight rise in protein.
Virus recoverable from throat swab or faeces.
Antibody-titre rise confirms the diagnosis retrospectively.

Treatment
1. Analgesic and anti-inflammatory drugs. Narcotics sometimes required.
2. Maintain respiration.

REFERENCE

POYNTON, F. J. (1943), *Lancet*, 2, 433.

POLYARTERITIS NODOSA

An uncommon disorder in which widespread focal panarteritis with fibrinoid necrosis of the vessel wall produces clinical involvement of many systems, in particular causing renal disease, heart failure, and peripheral neuropathy. The diagnosis is usually suggested by the association of arthritis and involvement of other systems and may be confirmed by biopsy.

Incidence

M. 4 : 1.

Any age (slight increase with age).

70 per cent have generalized muscle/joint pains at the onset of disease.

10 per cent have a chronic arthritis indistinguishable from rheumatoid arthritis at the time of onset of disease.

25 per cent have arthritis during the course of the disease; three types (*see* below).

1. *Acute type*. Transient migratory polyarthritis resembling that of rheumatic fever. Affects one or many joints often ankles, knees, shoulders, elbows, wrists, occasionally hands and feet. Resolves completely without deformity.
2. *Chronic type*. Chronic polyarthritis indistinguishable from rheumatoid arthritis (*see* p. 114).
3. *Pseudohypertrophic osteoarthropathy* (*see* p. 104) has been reported.

Course

Untreated, the disease is usually fatal within a year or two. 40 per cent survive 5 years with steroid therapy; prognosis worse with renal failure or hypertension.

Associations

1. Loss of weight, fever, and tachycardia (usual).
2. Renal disease (90 per cent). May present as chronic renal failure, acute renal failure with oedema and haematuria resembling acute glomerulonephritis (often without hypertension), or nephrotic syndrome.
3. Peripheral neuropathy (50 per cent). Either symmetrical sensorimotor type or mononeuritis multiplex.
4. Hypertension (50 per cent).
5. Heart failure or acute pericarditis (30 per cent). Myocardial infarction common and often painless.

6. Lung involvement (30 per cent). Bronchitis, asthma, or pneumonia may precede other systemic features by up to 10 years. Eosinophilia more common; hypertension and renal disease less common in this group.
7. Skin lesions (25 per cent). Purpura, bruising, peripheral gangrene, nodules, livedo reticularis.
8. Gastro-intestinal tract involvement. Abdominal pain, haemorrhage, rarely hepatitis at onset.
9. C.N.S. involvement. Organic psychosis, cerebral infarction.

XR

Acute type: normal.

Chronic type: changes of rheumatoid arthritis. Selective renal angiography may show arterial aneurysms.

Laboratory

Raised E.S.R.

Anaemia, leucocytosis (usual).

Eosinophilia (occasionally).

Proteinuria, haematuria, raised blood urea (common).

Positive latex test (20 per cent).

Raised gamma-globulin.

Australia antigen may be found.

Muscle biopsy positive in 40 per cent—choose tender area. Biopsy of other affected organs, e.g., kidney, should confirm. Biopsy of synovium shows either typical changes of polyarteritis or rheumatoid arthritis.

Treatment

Prednisolone 60 mg. daily; reduce slowly to maintenance dose, usually 10–30 mg. daily.

REFERENCES

BALL, J. (1954), *Annals of the Rheumatic Diseases*, **13**, 277.

LOVELL, R. R. H., and SCOTT, G. B. D. (1956), *Annals of the Rheumatic Diseases*, **15**, 46.

LOWMAN, E. W. (1952), *Annals of the Rheumatic Diseases*, **11**, 146.

ROX, G. A. (1957), *British Medical Journal*, **2**, 1148.

POLYMYALGIA RHEUMATICA

A not uncommon syndrome characterized by pains and stiffness in the shoulder and pelvic girdles.[1] Though patients complain of muscle pain, symptoms in fact arise from inflammation of joint capsules, tendons, and ligaments. In most cases the syndrome is not associated with any other disease. However, about 50 per cent of cases of temporal arteritis have symptoms identical to those of polymyalgia rheumatica, which usually precede the onset of headaches and ocular complications. Giant cell arteritis is found in both temporal arteritis and polymyalgia rheumatica and it is probable that the two diseases are different manifestations of the same pathological process. Rarely the polymyalgia rheumatica syndrome is the presenting feature of rheumatoid arthritis, malignant disease, or severe infections such as infective endocarditis.[2] May occasionally occur in pyrophosphate arthropathy (p. 108).

Incidence

F. 3 : 1.
Typical onset age 60+ but rarely 40+.
Joints always affected.

Joints affected

Sternoclavicular, acromioclavicular, shoulder, cervical spine, hips, and knees commonly.
Often lumbar spine.
Occasionally wrist and dorsal spine.
Small joint involvement is rare and should suggest rheumatoid arthritis.
Bilateral and symmetrical.
Central joints predominate.

Symptoms

Acute onset of severe pain and stiffness in muscles of shoulder and/or pelvic girdle.
Severe morning stiffness.
Malaise and weight-loss.

Signs

1. Limitation of movement of shoulders and/or hips (may disappear later in the day).
2. Tenderness of affected joints and surrounding soft tissue. Synovial thickening or joint effusion often found.
3. Arterial bruits occasionally.

Course

Spontaneous resolution usually within 2–4 years.
Respondes within days to corticosteroids.

Associations

Blindness is a rare complication of polymyalgia. However, an identical syndrome occurs in some cases of temporal arteritis in which blindness is not uncommon.

XR

Usually normal.
Changes of osteoarthritis are common in this age-group.

Laboratory

E.S.R. raised, usually over 50 mm. per hr.
5 per cent have normal E.S.R.
Temporal artery biopsy shows giant-cell arteritis in 20 per cent. Synovial biopsy shows non-specific synovitis.

Treatment

Prednisolone, initially 7·5–15 mg. daily. After a few months, reduce by 0·5–1·0 mg. daily each month. Continue smallest dose necessary to suppress all symptoms. Start treatment immediately on diagnosis. For temporal arteritis, use 40 mg. prednisolone daily or more if necessary.

REFERENCES

[1]BRUK, M. I. (1967), *Annals of the Rheumatic Diseases*, **26**, 103.

[2]HUSKISSON, E. C., and others (1977), *British Medical Journal*, **2**, 1459.

POLYMYOSITIS/DERMATOMYOSITIS

A connective-tissue disorder characterized by weakness particularly affecting proximal muscul-ature; histology shows necrosis of muscle, adjacent regeneration, and variable inflammatory change. The condition may be classified as follows: (1) *Polymyositis*, acute (with myoglobinuria), subacute, or chronic. 2. *Polymyositis with dominant muscular weakness* but with some evidence of associated collagen disease or dermatomyositis. (3) *Polymyositis complicating severe collagen disease*, or dermatomyositis with florid skin changes and minor muscle weakness. (4) *Polymyositis or dermatomyositis complicating malignant disease*. It is one of the features of mixed connective-tissue disease p. 75).

Incidence

F. 2 : 1.
Any age, peak 30–60 (15 per cent children).
Arthritis in 40 per cent; usually soon after onset of muscular symptoms, but rarely up to several years before.

Joints affected

Fingers (M.C.P. and P.I.P. joints) and wrists commonest.
Occasionally elbows, shoulders, knees, and ankles.
Bilateral and symmetrical.

Symptoms

Joint pains with morning stiffness.
Malaise and weight loss common.
Muscular weakness dominates the clinical picture, affecting proximal muscles, pelvic girdle first and most severely.
Muscle pain or tenderness present in 60 per cent.

Signs

Joints sometimes normal but more commonly swollen, warm, red, and tender.
Effusion often.
Restriction of movement usual.
Proximal muscle wasting, often not marked.

Course

Arthritis is transient, never deforming, and responds to steroids.
Muscle weakness progresses often with relapses and remissions.
30 per cent develop contractures.
15 per cent die of respiratory failure or infection.

Associations

1. Skin lesions (60 per cent): lilac-coloured facial rash in butterfly distribution, and on upper neck and limbs; often photo-sensitive, sometimes tender. May be accompanied by oedema especially in acute cases.
2. Dysphagia (50 per cent).
3. Raynaud's phenomenon (30 per cent).
4. Sjögren's syndrome and features of other collagen diseases (S.L.E., scleroderma, or polyarteritis nodosa) in 20 per cent.
5. Bursitis (occasionally).
6. Cancer (10 per cent)—commoner in those with dermatomyositis (20 per cent)—especially ovary, lung, breast, and stomach. Incidence increases with age—50 per cent over age 50.

XR

Joints normal.
Calcification of skin and proximal limb muscles especially in long-standing cases in young people.

Laboratory

E.S.R. raised in 50 per cent.
Serum aldolase raised in 75 per cent in active phase. Useful monitor of treatment.
Typical muscle biopsy in 75 per cent; others normal or non-specific.
E.M.G. usually abnormal but non-specific.
Latex test positive in 50 per cent; A.N.F. in 30 per cent.
L.E. cells usually negative.

Treatment

1. Prednisolone 60 mg. daily for 5 days, then 40 mg. daily. Reduce slowly to minimum maintenance (about 15 mg. daily). Arthritis resolves; muscles improve or resolve in 75 per cent. If no response, search for malignancy. Immuno-suppressives may be useful.
2. Physiotherapy to improve muscle function.

REFERENCES

BARWICK, D. D., and WALTON, J. N. (1963), *American Journal of Medicine*, **35**, 646.
LOGAN, R. G., and others (1966), *Annals of Internal Medicine*, **65**, 996.

PEARSON, C. M. (1959), *Arthritis and Rheumatism*, **2**, 127.

POST-SALMONELLA ARTHRITIS

A condition resembling Reiter's disease which follows *Salmonella* infection but is not due to the presence of the organism in the joint. It has been described after infection with *Salmonella typhimurium* but probably occurs less commonly with other types of *Salmonella*.

Incidence
M. = F.
Age 10–50.
2·5 per cent of cases of infection with *Salmonella typhimurium*.
1 to 2 weeks after onset of fever and diarrhoea.

Joints affected
Polyarticular.
Knee (60 per cent) or ankle (60 per cent) usually affected.
Occasionally also wrist, hand, cervical spine, or big toe.
Often migratory; usually asymmetrical.

Symptoms
Pain and swelling.

Signs
Soft-tissue swelling and tenderness.
Joints occasionally red and warm with effusion.
Fever usual.

Course
Chronic with remissions and relapses, lasting up to 6 months, but eventually resolving completely without sequelae.

Associations
1. Diarrhoea preceding arthritis.
2. Other features of Reiter's disease, conjunctivitis, iritis, or urethritis, are rarely found.

XR
Normal.

Laboratory
Raised E.S.R.
Positive agglutination test for *Salmonella*; rising titre. Organism may be isolated from stools but not from joint fluid.

Treatment
1. Analgesic and anti-inflammatory drugs.
2. Antibiotics should be given but have no effect on arthritis.

REFERENCE

VARTIAINEN, J., and HURRI, L. (1964), *Acta Medica Scandinavica*, **175**, 771.

PSEUDOHYPERTROPHIC OSTEOARTHROPATHY
(Pachydermoperiostitis; Marie-Bamberger syndrome)

The syndrome of digital clubbing, swelling of the distal parts of the limbs, periostitis, synovitis, and thickening of facial skin. It may be due to: (1) *Benign or malignant, primary or secondary tumours of lung, pleura, heart, diaphragm, mediastinum, or upper gastro-intestinal tract.* (2) *Pulmonary suppuration* (bronchiectasis, lung abscess, empyema). (3) *Aortic aneurysm.* (4) *Gastro-intestinal disorder*: ulcerative colitis, Crohn's disease, steatorrhoea; cirrhosis of the liver. (5) *Cyanotic congenital heart disease.* (6) Rarely, the condition is inherited as an *autosomal dominant.*

Incidence

M. 5 : 1.
Commonest in middle-aged men with bronchial carcinoma.
Occurs in 5 per cent of cases of bronchial carcinoma; may precede other manifestations by several months. Occurs in 50 per cent of cases of pleural and diaphragmatic tumour. Rare in other conditions.
In non-malignant conditions, the syndrome follows years after the development of the primary condition.
Hereditary type appears after puberty.

Joints affected

Knees, wrists, ankles, elbows, and M.C.P. joints.
Others rare.
Usually bilateral and symmetrical affecting all four limbs; unilateral and confined to upper limb with Pancoast syndrome and aortic aneurysm.

Symptoms

Sudden onset of pain, often severe, deep, and burning, in affected joints.
Weakness; morning stiffness; sweating of hands and feet.
Insidious onset with non-malignant conditions.

Signs

Joints are swollen with painful limitation of movement.
Overlying skin may be warm, dusky, red, and thickened; effusion common; marked tenderness of distal ends of long bones is characteristic.
Fever occasionally.

Course

Remissions and relapses coincide with changes in underlying disease; eradication cures.
Prognosis determined by underlying disease.

Associations

1. Clubbing (always); facial thickening resembling acromegaly (occasionally).
2. Features of underlying disease.

XR

Periosteal elevation along the shafts of the long bones, starting at the distal end, spreading proximally. Later osteoporosis and sometimes tufting of distal phalanges of hands.

Laboratory

Raised E.S.R. in active phase.
Synovial fluid: non-inflammatory; W.B.C. $< 2000 \times 10^9$/dl.; predominantly mononuclears.

Treatment

1. Appropriate treatment of the underlying disorders produces rapid remission. Prolonged search for neoplasm may be required.
2. Vagotomy may help if thoracotomy reveals inoperable malignancy.
3. Analgesic and anti-inflammatory drugs; steroids or ACTH sometimes useful.

REFERENCES

BERMAN, B. (1963), *Archives of Internal Medicine*, **112**, 947.

MENDLOWITZ, M. (1942), *Medicine*, **21**, 269.

PSEUDOXANTHOMA ELASTICUM

A rare genetic disorder inherited as an autosomal recessive, and caused by a defect in elastic tissue. It is characterized by thickened, leathery, lax skin particularly of the neck, angioid streaking of the fundus of the eye and peripheral arterial disease. Arthritis is not usually a feature, but intermittent pain, tenderness and swelling of one or more joints has been described. Each episode lasted for weeks or months and resolved completely without residua.

REFERENCE

Sairanen, E., and others (1970), *Acta Rheumatologica Scandinavica*, **160**, 130.

PSITTACOSIS

Infection by *Chlamydia psittaci* usually causes atypical pneumonia but a migratory polyarthritis is an occasional complication. The infection is usually acquired from parrots or less commonly poultry, pigeons, canaries or other birds. After an incubation period of 1–3 weeks, the patient becomes acutely febrile with malaise, headache, muscle pains and a dry cough. Chest X-ray shows pneumonitis and may vary from day to day. The diagnosis is usually confirmed only in retrospect by a rising titre of antibodies. Prognosis—variable. Severe pneumonitis may prove fatal. Arthritis is transient. Because of its migratory nature, it may closely resemble rheumatic fever. *Treatment:* Tetracycline 500 mg. q.d.s.

REFERENCE

Simpson, R. W., and others (1971), *British Medical Journal*, **1**, 694.

PSORIASIS

A very common skin disease characterized by the presence of well-defined, dry, raised, red, scaly patches, not itchy, particularly on the extensor surfaces of the knees and elbows and on the scalp.

Incidence

M. = F.
Usual age of onset 20–50.
10 per cent develop psoriatic arthropathy.
Psoriasis may be minimal or absent and usually precedes arthritis often by many years.
Rarely arthritis precedes skin disease.
Occasionally exacerbations of psoriasis and arthritis coincide.
30 per cent give a family history of psoriasis.

Joints affected

Polyarticular.
Small joints of hands predominate (70 per cent).
Four patterns, but many compound and intermediate varieties.
1. *Distal type* (55 per cent). Affects distal interphalangeal joints, often P.I.P. joints and occasionally others.
2. *Seronegative indistinguishable type* (35 per cent). Joint involvement is clinically indistinguishable from rheumatoid arthritis; affects hands, feet, wrists, shoulders, elbows, knees, and ankles. Symmetrical.
3. *Deforming type* (10 per cent). Affects D.I.P., P.I.P., and M.C.P. joints of hands, wrists, elbows, shoulders, knees, and toes commonly; often cervical spine and ankle. Causes opera-glass hand or foot (arthritis mutilans).
4. *Spondylitis*. 10 per cent of patients with psoriatic arthropathy have ankylosing spondylitis, usually in association with the peripheral arthritis of psoriasis. This is not particularly a condition of the male sex.

Symptoms

Onset either acute or chronic.
Pain seldom prominent except in deforming type.
Morning stiffness unusual.

PSORIASIS (*continued*)

Signs
Acute stage: red, hot, swollen joint (sausage digit resembling gout).
Chronic stage: swollen joints, erythema often marked.

Course
Recurrent or progressive, but often mild except in the deforming type in which rapid progression to severe deformities is usual.

Associations
1. Nail changes (hyperkeratosis or pitting) in 80 per cent of patients with arthritis and 10 per cent without.
2. Hyperuricaemia in 30 per cent.
3. Tendon-sheath effusions rare (5 per cent). No nodules.

XR
1. Erosions.
2. Sclerosis of joint margins.
3. Proliferation of bone.
4. Cysts.
5. Ankylosis.
6. Destruction of bone ends in deforming type.
7. 'Mushrooming' (impaction of the distal end of one phalanx in the base of the next).
8. 30 per cent have sacro-iliitis.
9. Rarely paravertebral ossification.[2]

Laboratory
E.S.R. normal except in acute stage.
Latex test negative.

Treatment
1. Analgesic and anti-inflammatory drugs.
2. Azathioprine for severe cases.
3. Gold may be useful but is less effective than in rheumatoid arthritis.
Avoid systemic steroids. Antimalarials contra-indicated (risk of exfoliative dermatitis).

REFERENCES
[1] BAKER, H., and others (1963), *Annals of Internal Medicine*, **58**, 909.
[2] BYWATERS, E. G. L., and DIXON, A. ST. J. (1965), *Annals of the Rheumatic Diseases*, **24**, 313.
[3] WRIGHT, V. (1959), *American Journal of Medicine*, **27**, 454.

PSYCHOGENIC RHEUMATISM

A common condition in which joint pain arises from psychological disturbance. This may be associated with various psychiatric conditions, particularly anxiety states and depression, but rarely hysteria.

Incidence
F. 3 : 1.
Any age, particularly 30–60.
Commonest in the lower social classes; often obsessional, aggressive, and resentful people with a F.H. of neurotic illness; emotional stress may precede onset of symptoms.

Joints affected
Any or all.
Low-back pain common.
Non-dominant side commoner than dominant. Site may be determined by hysterical conversion phenomena, e.g., to immobilize a limb.

Symptoms
Pain and stiffness; pain is often described in vivid terms, e.g., searing, and may be continuous with no variation in severity and no response to rest or analgesics.

Signs
None.

Course
Chronic, with recurrent visits to specialists until the correct diagnosis is made.

Associations
1. Numerous other complaints particularly headache, tension, depression, and sleeplessness. History of many previous illnesses and investigations.
2. Underlying psychiatric states (*see above*).

XR
Normal.
Beware of minor degenerative changes.

Laboratory
Unhelpful.

E.S.R. normal.
Beware of weakly positive latex test, anti-nuclear factor, or elevated serum uric acid which may lead to an incorrect diagnosis.

Treatment

1. Make a positive diagnosis and reassure the patient firmly but tactfully. Avoid diagnostic uncertainty, repeated visits to hospital, numerous investigations, and therapeutic vacillation.
2. Treatment depends on underlying psychiatric state: diazepam 2 mg. t.d.s. especially for anxiety; imipramine 25 mg. t.d.s. especially for depression; amitriptyline 50–100 mg. *nocte* for sleeplessness. Simple analgesics such as paracetamol.
3. Discussion of the problems which have caused the illness may be helpful.

REFERENCE

ELLMAN, P., and SHAW, D. (1950), *Annals of the Rheumatic Diseases*, **9**, 341.

PYODERMA GANGRENOSUM

A rare skin disease characterized by chronic ulceration of the legs. The ulcers are irregular in outline with a ragged edge and necrotic base. They increase in size slowly, reaching a diameter of up to 10 cm. They are chronic but of variable duration, from weeks to years. There may be one or many, on the lower legs, thighs, buttocks or trunks. Pyoderma gangrenosum may be associated with various systemic diseases including ulcerative colitis, myeloma or paraproteinaemia, rheumatoid arthritis and paroxysmal nocturnal haemoglobinuria. There may also be a progressive seronegative erosive polyarthritis:

Incidence
Arthritis is common (about 50 per cent of all cases)—may precede or follow skin disease and bears no relation to activity of skin disease.

Joints affected
Many joints as in rheumatoid arthritis, but prominent involvement of D.I.P. and first C.M.C. joints.
Bilateral and symmetrical.

Symptoms
Pain and stiffness of affected joints.

Signs
Joints are swollen and may show other signs of inflammation such as warmth.

Course
Slowly progressive joint destruction—over the years deformities develop like those of rheumatoid arthritis.

Associations
Other conditions may be associated with pyoderma gangrenosum (*see above*). No systemic vasculitis, nodules or other extra-articular features of rheumatoid.

XR
Erosions, porosis, loss of joint space.
Sacro-iliitis occasionally.

Laboratory
Latex and A.N.F.: negative.
HLA B27: negative.
Synovial fluid: inflammatory with raised W.B.C. predominantly neutrophils.
Low complement.
Synovial biopsy: similar to rheumatoid arthritis.

Treatment
Symptomatic: analgesic-anti-inflammatory drugs.

REFERENCE

HOLT, P., and others (1977), *Annals of Rheumatic Diseases*, **36**, 285.

PYROPHOSPHATE ARTHROPATHY

A condition associated with deposition of crystals of calcium pyrophosphate dihydrate (CPPD) into joints. There are several different patterns of disease:[1] 1. Acute attacks of self-limiting arthritis ('pseudogout')—about 25 per cent of cases present in this way. 2. The commonest manifestation is a chronic polyarthritis indistinguishable from osteoarthritis ('pseudo-osteoarthritis'). There may be superimposed attacks of pseudogout. This disease is distinguished from osteoarthritis by the linear calcification of cartilage ('spotty' in osteoarthritis, see p. 90) and by the nature of the crystals. About 50 per cent of cases follow this pattern. 3. A recurrent low-grade seronegative polyarthritis ('pseudo-rheumatoid arthritis') occurs in about 5 per cent of cases. Episodes lasts for months but resolve completely. There is morning stiffness and joint effusions which add to the confusion. A severe familial variety has been described but is rare. 4. A severe destructive arthritis may occur and resembles Charcot joints ('pseudoneurotrophic joints'), usually affecting knees, hips or ankles. 5. An acute spinal syndrome may occur resembling an acute disc prolapse[2] and in severe polyarticular cases, a stiff spine resembling ankylosing spondylitis has been described. 6. Polymyalgia rheumatica may rarely occur[2]. Different syndromes may occur at the same or different times in the same patient. The term *chondrocalcinosis articularis* should be reserved for the radiological appearance of linear cartilage calcification.

Incidence

M. = F.

Age 30 + .

Typical onset age 60 (but earlier in familial cases).

Joints affected

Knee commonest.

Often hips, ankles, shoulders, elbows, and wrists.

Occasionally toes and fingers. Rarely affects big toe resembling gout, or spine.

Usually one joint in acute attacks.

Chronic type affects many joints symmetrically as in osteoarthritis.

Symptoms

Pain and stiffness.

Sudden onset in acute type; may be precipitated by surgery or trauma.

Signs

Acute: red, hot, swollen joint; effusion usual.
Chronic: bony swelling resembling osteoarthritis. Effusions common.

Course

Acute attacks last weeks or months and recur at irregular intervals.

Chronic type is slowly progressive with outcome resembling osteoarthritis.

Associations

Most cases have no abnormality of serum calcium, iron or alkaline phosphatase. The following are unusual associations:

1. Hypercalcaemia, particularly primary hyperparathyroidism but also malignancy and other causes.

2. Haemochromatosis.

3. Hypophosphatasia[3].

XR

Affected joints show linear calcification of cartilage and degenerative changes indistinguishable from those of osteoarthritis. Calcification is usually seen in knees and wrists. Other joints such as the hips may show severe osteoarthritis without calcification.

Laboratory

Raised E.S.R. and leucocytosis in acute attacks.

Synovial fluid: brick-shaped crystals which are weakly positively birefringent. Usually found in pseudogout and in about 50 per cent of chronic cases. W.B.C. about $10,000 \times 10^9$/dl. in pseudogout, mainly polymorphs; about 3000 in pseudo-osteoarthritis, mainly monocytes.

Most cases have normal serum calcium. Always check.

Treatment

Acute stage:

1. Aspiration of affected joints. Inject with prednisolone.

2. Indomethacin or other anti-inflammatory drugs.

3. Rest.

Effects variable and sometimes disappointing

Chronic type:

As for osteoarthritis (*see* p. 90).

REFERENCES

[1]McCarty, D. J. (1975), *Bulletin on Rheumatic Diseases*, **25**, 804.

[2]Storey, G. O., and Huskisson, E. C. (1977), *British Medical Journal*, **2**, 21.

[3]O'Duffy, J. D. (1970), *Arthritis and Rheumatism*, **13**, 381.

[4]McCarty, D. J., and others (1963), *Annals of Internal Medicine*, **56**, 711.

[5]McCarty, D. J., and Hollander, J. L. (1961), *Annals of Internal Medicine*, **54**, 452.

[6]Zitnan, D., and Sitaj, S. (1963), *Annals of the Rheumatic Diseases*, **22**, 142.

RAT-BITE FEVER

Infection with *Streptobacillus moniliformis* (Haverhill fever) or *Spirillum minus*, acquired either from the bite of an infected rat, mouse, or other rodent, or ingestion of food or milk contaminated by rat excreta. Incubation period is about 1 week for *Str. moniliformis* (1–14 days) and about 2 weeks for *S. minus* (5–28 days). The rat bite often appears to be healing when there is a sudden appearance of fever with an influenza-like illness; the rat bite becomes inflamed and there is a local lymphadenopathy. The disease is particularly found in North America and Japan, but may occur anywhere.

Incidence

M. = F.

Any age.

Arthritis is common in *Streptobacillus* infection, but rare in *Spirillum* infection.

Joints affected

Polyarticular.

Affects knees, shoulders, elbows, wrists, and small joints of hands.

Unilateral or bilateral.

Symptoms

Acute onset of pain, usually severe.

Signs

Sometimes none.

Sometimes effusion with marked tenderness.

Course

Arthritis resolves completely with early and effective therapy.

Untreated, the bouts of fever may recur for up to 17 years.

Associations

1. Recurrent bouts of fever, each lasting a few days and occurring about once per week. Nausea, headache, and rigors.
2. Generalized erythematous rash, sometimes with pustules.
3. Lymphadenopathy and splenomegaly with *Spirillum* infection.
4. Other complications are myositis and endocarditis.

XR

Normal.

Laboratory

Leucocytosis.

Raised E.S.R.

Streptobacillus: culture of wound, synovial fluid or blood.

Spirillum: smear or guinea-pig inoculation of material from the bite or a lymph-node.

Treatment

1. Penicillin and streptomycin. Intra-articular administration unnecessary.
2. Aspiration of effusions, repeated if necessary.

REFERENCE

McGill, R. C., and others (1966), *British Medical Journal*, 1, 1213.

REITER'S DISEASE

The triad of arthritis, urethritis, and conjunctivitis which usually follows non-specific (non-gonococcal) urethritis, or less commonly, cystitis or prostatitis, the genital type. In some parts of the world (Scandinavia, North Africa, Asia) the triad follows dysentery or occasionally non-specific diarrhoea, the intestinal type.

Incidence

M. 20 : 1.
Usual age of onset 20–40.
Complicates 0·8 per cent of cases of urethral infection in males, occurring up to about 4 weeks after sexual exposure, which is commonly promiscuous.
Complicates 0·2 per cent of cases of dysentery occurring usually 10–30 days, but rarely up to 3 months after intestinal manifestations.

Joints affected

Knee (90 per cent) and ankle (75 per cent) commonest.
Feet often (40 per cent).
Shoulder, wrist, elbow, hip and spine (30 per cent).
Polyarticular (90 per cent).
Asymmetrical (75 per cent).
Rarely migratory.

Symptoms

Acute onset of joint pain and swelling, dysuria, and penile discharge.
Onset occasionally insidious.
Pain in the heel in 30 per cent.

Signs

Red, hot, tender joints in acute stage; occasionally localized spinal tenderness.
Pyrexia (60 per cent).

Course

First attack usually resolves within 6 months; rarely becomes chronic.
50 per cent relapse, not usually associated with sexual exposure, urethritis, or dysentery.
20 per cent have continued relapsing or chronic arthritis with attacks recurring at irregular intervals, weeks or months apart, causing disability but seldom deformity.
30 per cent develop spondylitis, usually mild, with X-ray changes localized to small areas of the spine or sacro-iliac joints. 60 per cent of these patients also have involvement of hips, knees, ankles, or feet, usually monarticular.

Associations

Acute stage:
1. Urethritis usual.
2. Conjunctivitis (30 per cent).
3. Circinate balanitis (25 per cent).
4. Keratoderma blenorrhagica (15 per cent).
5. Tenosynovitis, usually Achilles tendon (20 per cent).
6. Plantar fasciitis (20 per cent).
7. Keratitis (5 per cent).
Late:
1. Iritis (10 per cent)—commoner in those with chronic or recurring arthritis (40 per cent). Unilateral.
2. Cardiac conduction defects and aortic incompetence (rare).

XR

Early: normal.
Late:
1. Sacro-iliitis (30 per cent), usually bilateral.
2. Localized spinal changes of ankylosing spondylitis (15 per cent).
3. 'Fluffy' periosteal new bone formation particularly around the wrists, ankles, or pelvis. Calcaneal spur in 10 per cent.
4. Rarely joint erosions or ankylosis.

Laboratory

Raised E.S.R. in acute stage.
Latex test negative.
Joint fluid: inflammatory.
Raised complement level.
Gonococcus found in genital tract in up to 50 per cent but not from blood or joint fluid.
Tissue antigen HLA B27 (75 per cent).

Treatment

Rest in acute stage.
Analgesic and anti-inflammatory drugs.
Aspiration and steroid injection.

REFERENCES

Genital type
CSONKA, G. W. (1958), *British Medical Journal*, **1**, 1088.
MASON, R. M., and others (1959), *Journal of Bone and Joint Surgery*, **41B**, 137.
WRIGHT, V. (1963), *Annals of the Rheumatic Diseases*, **22**, 77.

Intestinal type
PARONEN, I. (1948), *Acta Medica Scandinavica*, supplement 212.
SAIRANEN, E., and others (1969), *Acta Medica Scandinavica*, **185**, 57.

RELAPSING POLYCHONDRITIS

A rare non-hereditary condition characterized by inflammation of cartilage in several sites, including external ears, nose, and joints.

Two types of arthritis occur: more common (75 per cent) is an episodic migratory asymmetrical non-deforming polyarthritis. Occasionally (25 per cent) there is a chronic symmetrical polyarthritis resembling rheumatoid arthritis but seronegative. This may be progressive and destructive.

Incidence

M.=F.
Onset typically about age 40 (2–80).
Arthritis in 80 per cent, often a presenting feature or early in the disease.

Joints affected

Small joints of hands, knees, and ankles commonest.
Any other joint may be involved.
Spine and sacro-iliac joints affected later.
Either asymmetrical, migratory and episodic or chronic bilateral and symmetrical.

Symptoms

Pain.
Morning stiffness.

Signs

Joints are swollen and tender with limitation of movement. Effusions occasionally.
Costochondral junctions and xiphoid process may be swollen and tender.

Course

Attacks of cartilage inflammation recur at variable intervals, sometimes with remissions lasting years.
Episodes of arthritis are not related in time to episodes of chondritis. They occur at irregular intervals several times each year and last for days or weeks, resolving without deformity. Some chronic cases are progressive and develop severe deformities and disability.
A few cases progress rapidly to death from tracheal or bronchial obstruction.

Associations

1. 80 per cent have episodes of pain in nose or external ear which become red, tender, and swollen. Eventually the cartilage gets soft and flabby. Saddle-nose deformity, epistaxis, or rhinorrhoea common. Deafness occasionally (middle-ear involvement).
2. 50 per cent have episcleritis, conjunctivitis, or iritis.
3. Occasionally involvement of larynx (respiratory difficulty may require tracheotomy), trachea, or bronchi.

XR

Often normal.
Loss of joint space; degenerative changes.

Laboratory

Anaemia and raised E.S.R. in active phases.
Latex test occasionally positive.
Biopsy of cartilage: inflammatory changes, cartilage necrosis, and replacement with fibrous tissue.
Synovial fluid: viscous; few cells.

Treatment

1. Salicylates and other non-steroidal anti-inflammatory drugs, steroids, or ACTH in active phases. Low dose of steroids may prevent attacks.
2. Avoid trauma and surgery to affected areas.

REFERENCES

KAYE, R. L., and SONES, D. A. (1964), *Annals of Internal Medicine*, **60**, 653.
O'HANLON, M., and others (1976), *Arthritis and Rheumatism*, **19**, 191.

THOULD, A. K., and others (1965), *Annals of the Rheumatic Diseases*, **24**, 563.

RENAL TRANSPLANTATION

After renal transplantation,[1] 30 per cent of patients develop arthritis, usually in the first year after operation. The following varieties occur:

1. *Pyrophosphate Arthropathy* (*see* p. 108).

2. *Avascular Necrosis* (*see* p. 10), due to high-dose steroid therapy.

3. *Opportunistic Infection and Septic Arthritis* (*see* p. 123) due to immune suppression.

4. '*Osteogenic*' *Synovitis* due to hyperparathyroidism (*see* p. 54).

5. *Calcium Phosphate* (*Apatite*) *Deposition around Joints* occurs after transplantation and also in patients on *chronic dialysis.*[2] This gives rise to episodes of acute arthritis resembling those of pyrophosphate arthropathy, particularly affecting the small joints of the hands, sometimes wrists, shoulders, or elbows and rarely knees or big toes. Attacks are usually monarticular but occasionally several joints of one limb are affected, e.g., elbow, wrist, and hand. There is a sudden onset of severe pain and affected joints are warm, red, swollen, and very tender. Tender 'pseudotophi' form around the affected joints and after a number of attacks the hands may resemble the advanced stage of tophaceous gout; the condition is distinguished from pyrophosphate arthropathy by the nature of the deposit which has the characteristics of apatite. XR shows calcified deposits. Calcium levels are often low, but phosphate levels are high and the calcium phosphate product is always raised. Anti-inflammatory drugs are useful for the acute attack.

6. *Arthralgia* or non-specific acute or chronic synovitis, for which no cause can be found, has also been described. Some of these cases may have early avascular necrosis and they should therefore be immobilized.

The latex test is commonly positive after renal transplantation regardless of the presence or absence of arthritis, and anti-DNA antibodies are often found. Hyperuricaemia is common and parallels changes in blood urea.

REFERENCES

[1] *British Medical Journal* (1967), **3**, 323.

[2] CANER, J. E. Z., and DECKER, J. L. (1964), *American Journal of Medicine*, **36**, 571.

Haemodialysis

Patients with chronic renal failure on regular haemodialysis are also liable to develop *pyrophosphate arthropathy, hyperparathyroidism*, and *calcium phosphate deposition around joints* (*see above*). In some centres a variety of bone disease ('Newcastle bone disease') is common in such patients, beginning between 6 months and 4 years after the start of dialysis. They complain of pains, usually in the feet and ankles but sometimes in the knees, groins, ribs, shoulders, and back. There may also be acute painful episodes due to pathological fracture of ribs, femoral neck, or spine. Associated features include kyphosis, loss of height, and proximal muscular weakness and wasting. XR shows porosis, especially in the hands, either periarticular or in a patchy distribution in the shafts of the metacarpals and phalanges. There may be fractures, pseudofractures, and occasionally changes of hyperparathyroidism. There are no consistent biochemical abnormalities and the condition does not respond to vitamin D. Treatment: analgesics.

REFERENCE

SIMPSON, W., and others (1972), *Proceedings of the Royal Society of Medicine*, **65**, 477.

RHEUMATIC FEVER

An acute febrile illness characterized by arthritis, carditis, and chorea, which follows strepto-coccal infection. It has become less frequent and less severe in the United Kingdom but is still common in some other parts of the world. Its importance lies in the development of chronic rheumatic heart disease as a possible sequel.

Incidence

M. = F.
Peak age 5–15; rare below age 3 and above age 20.
Arthritis in 80 per cent; arthralgia in 10 per cent; usually a presenting feature.

Joints affected

Polyarticular.
Knees (75 per cent) and ankles (50 per cent) commonest.
Occasionally elbows, wrists, hips, and small joints of feet (25 per cent).
Rarely shoulders and small joints of hands (10 per cent).
Usually transient and flitting from joint to joint—only one or two joints affected at one time.
25 per cent monarticular.

Symptoms

Joint pain and swelling.
History of sore throat about 2 weeks previously.

Signs

Joints are usually hot, red, tender, and swollen.
Effusions occur in large joints.
Fever (90 per cent), usually sustained.

Course

Single joint seldom involved for more than a few days. Arthritis abates within a few weeks but may be more persistent in adults than children.
No residua except very rarely Jaccoud's syndrome (see p. 60).
Prognosis depends on cardiac involvement.
Primary carditis rare in adults; almost certain in second or third attacks in children.

Associations

1. Carditis (40 per cent): pericarditis (rub), pericardial effusion, myocarditis (tachy-cardia, heart failure), endocarditis (murmurs). Signs usually develop in the first week of the illness.
2. Subcutaneous nodules (10 per cent).
3. Chorea (10 per cent).
4. Erythema marginatum (5 per cent); rarely erythema nodosum.

XR

Normal.
CXR shows cardiac enlargement in 20 per cent.

Laboratory

Raised E.S.R. (90 per cent).
Throat swab: group A β-haemolytic strepto-cocci in 25 per cent.
A.S.O. titre raised in 75 per cent.
Raised LDH with carditis.
E.C.G.: conduction disturbance, signs of pericarditis or myocarditis.

Treatment

1. Bed-rest probably wise in the presence of active carditis.
2. Salicylates used to give symptomatic relief. There is no evidence that steroids prevent development of chronic valve disease.
3. Penicillin should be given in the acute phase to eliminate streptococci and later to prevent recurrence. Consider tonsillectomy.
4. Treatment of complications, e.g., heart failure with digitalis and diuretics.

REFERENCE

FEINSTEIN, A. R., and SPAGNUOLO, M. (1962), *Medicine*, **41**, 279.

RHEUMATOID ARTHRITIS

A common and widespread chronic polyarthritis characterized by bilateral symmetrical joint involvement, erosions on X-ray, positive tests for rheumatoid factor, and pathologically a chronic proliferative synovitis with villous hypertrophy, infiltration of lymphocytes and plasma cells, and lymphoid nodules. Diagnostic criteria are available.[2]

Incidence

6 per cent of females; 2 per cent of males; world-wide.
Onset age 16–70, commonest 20–55.

Joints affected

Initially polyarticular in 75 per cent affecting small joints of hands or feet (60 per cent), large joints (30 per cent), or both (5 per cent). 25 per cent monarticular affecting knee most commonly (50 per cent), sometimes shoulder, wrist, or hip (40 per cent), ankle or elbow (10 per cent), small joints rarely.

Ultimately affects hands (P.I.P. joints in 85 per cent, M.C.P. in 70 per cent, D.I.P. in 30 per cent) and wrists (80 per cent) predominantly.
Commonly knees (80 per cent).
Often ankles (70 per cent), shoulders (60 per cent), M.T.P. joints and toes (60 per cent), elbows (50 per cent), cervical spine (50 per cent), and hips (40 per cent).
Temporomandibular joints affected transiently in 50 per cent.
Rarely crico-arytenoid joints.
Usually bilateral and symmetrical eventually.

Symptoms

Insidious onset of joint pains and stiffness.
15 per cent start with an acute arthritis.
Generalized morning stiffness usual, lasting up to 6 hours.
Often accompanied by general ill health, fatigue, and weight-loss, which may precede joint symptoms by a few months.

Signs

1. Affected joints are usually swollen and tender with limitation of movement. Swelling due to effusion (40 per cent) or synovial thickening in early cases and to bony overgrowth in late 'burnt-out' cases.
2. Signs of acute inflammation such as warmth (20 per cent) and erythema (10 per cent) particularly in early stages and with exacerbations.
3. Muscle wasting around affected joints.

Special Features of Individual Joints

Hands: ulnar deviation at M.C.P. joints develops between 1 and 5 years after onset. Less common are boutonnière (flexion at P.I.P. joint) and swan-neck (hyper-extension at P.I.P. joint) deformities of fingers. Rarely there is arthritis mutilans with *main-en-lorgnette* (opera-glass hand) due to bone destruction and soft-tissue excess.
Wrist: prominent tender ulnar styloid process, with pain on pronation/supination.
Knees: Baker's cyst (cystic swelling in popliteal fossa) common. Flexion or valgus deformity and instability may occur later.
Feet:[3] tender prominent metatarsal heads with secondary corns; lateral deviation and overriding of toes with pressure sores.
Cervical spine: atlanto-axial subluxation (*see* **XR**) present in 30 per cent of hospital cases causing pain and very rarely spinal cord compression or vertebral artery occlusion.
Crico-arytenoid joint involvement causes hoarseness, stridor, dyspnoea, dysphagia, and recurrent bronchitis; sedatives dangerous; tracheostomy occasionally required.

Course

1. *Episodic* (25 per cent): average patient of this type has three attacks of arthritis, one every 2 years (very variable, may be up to 15 years), each lasting about 6 months. This group merges with palindromic rheumatism (*see* p. 94) in which the attacks are much shorter. Many cases eventually develop persistent arthritis.
2. *Persistent*: chronic arthritis with partial remissions and exacerbations. The mon-articular type remains monarticular in 60 per cent; the other 40 per cent develop polyarthritis in up to 10 years. Of the 25 per cent with initially unilateral involvement 90 per cent become bilateral and symmetrical within 2 years. Individual joints once involved, usually remain involved, though activity fluctuates. Joints tend to become 'burnt out' (inactive) after many years, and in this stage resemble advanced osteo-arthritic joints. Ultimately 50 per cent of patients have little or no disability; 40 per cent have some disability and 10 per cent are completely disabled.

RHEUMATOID ARTHRITIS (*continued*)

Nonarticular Manifestations:[4,5]

Periarticular Soft Tissues

1. Nodules (20 per cent) usually below elbows but almost anywhere else.
2. Tenosynovitis[6] around hands or wrists (65 per cent) causing pain, local swelling, tenderness, trigger finger, dysfunction, and flexion deformity.
3. Bursitis (common), particularly olecranon, causes swelling and discomfort.
4. Synovial cysts appear around any joint but particularly posterior to the knee (Baker's cyst). Raised pressure in knees with large effusions forces fluid into the cyst and may also cause joint rupture with calf pain, ankle oedema, and positive Homan's sign resembling deep-vein thrombosis.
5. Muscle wasting.
6. Ligamentous laxity leads to hypermobility and deformities, particularly important in causing ulnar deviation and atlanto-axial subluxation.

Skin

1. Tight, wasted skin common over finger-tips (not unlike scleroderma).
2. Leg ulcers (rarely), due to trauma (especially in patients on steroids), hypostasis, or associated with vasculitis and Felty's syndrome.

Eyes

1. Scleritis, episcleritis, and scleromalacia perforans—rare, but may lead to loss of vision.
2. Sjögren's syndrome[7] (15 per cent): dry eyes and mouth; confirm by Schirmer's test or Rose Bengal staining; associated with high incidence of allergic reaction, hyperglobulinaemia, auto-antibodies, etc.

Heart

1. Granulomatous lesions in myocardium and valves (rarely cause heart failure), valve lesions (particularly aortic incompetence), and mural thrombi with embolism.
2. Pericarditis; rub audible at some time in about 10 per cent; rarely constrictive.

Vasculitis

Skin lesions around finger nails in 5 per cent; rarely gangrene of fingers or toes.

Neuropathy

1. Compression; carpal tunnel syndrome (50 per cent) shortly before or after onset of arthritis. (*See also* p. 23.)
2. Symmetrical sensorimotor (5 per cent) usually affecting legs.
3. Digital: patchy sensory loss over tips of fingers and toes.
4. Autonomic (rare).

Lymphadenopathy (30 per cent)
And **splenomegaly** (rare).

Lung involvement[8]

1. Fibrosing alveolitis (rare).
2. Pleural effusion: 8 per cent of men; may be the presenting feature of rheumatoid arthritis. Fluid may have low glucose; positive latex test or 'rheumatoid' cells suggestive but not diagnostic.
3. Nodules in lungs or pleura.
4. Caplan's syndrome (multiple pulmonary nodules on chest X-ray in coal workers, iron-foundry workers, etc.).
5. Increased incidence of small airway obstruction in smokers.
6. Rarely acute pneumonitis.

Anaemia

Common and proportional to disease activity. Multiple causation includes failure of marrow iron utilization ('anaemia of infection') and aspirin.
Felty's syndrome:[9] splenomegaly and leucopenia; infections common.

Infections[10]

Joints commonest site; *Staphylococcus aureus* commonest organism; may be silent, and not always accompanied by fever or leucocytosis.

Oedema

1. Localized chronic oedema of one hand or forearm (rare).
2. Ankle oedema (10 per cent) with active disease.

Osteoporosis and fractures

Aggravated by steroid therapy; important cause of sudden worsening of pain in one joint.

Amyloidosis

Presents as proteinuria; may progress to renal failure.
Diagnosis by rectal, fat, or renal biopsy.

RHEUMATOID ARTHRITIS (*continued*)

XR
Early:
1. Periarticular osteoporosis.
2. Erosions. Changes best seen in X-rays of hands and feet.

Late:
1. Loss of joint space.
2. Bone destruction.
3. Rarely ankylosis.

Special Sites
Cervical spine. Ask for views in flexion and extension; any increase in the distance between the odontoid process and the anterior arch of the atlas in flexion is abnormal and indicates atlanto-axial subluxation.

Hip. Head of femur appears to 'burrow' into the acetabulum and may progress to protrusio acetabuli. Note also absence of sclerosis (cf. osteoarthritis).

Laboratory
Anaemia and raised E.S.R. common with active disease.
Latex test positive in 80 per cent (Rose-Waaler in 60 per cent).
A.N.F. often positive.
L.E. cells present in 10 per cent but never anti-DNA antibodies.
Synovial fluid: often appears purulent (yellow or green and turbid). Low viscosity. W.B.C. up to 100,000 $\times$ 10^9/dl.; mostly neutrophils. Latex test parallels serum titre and has no diagnostic significance in sero-negative cases. Sterile on culture.
Synovial biopsy may show non-specific chronic synovitis or characteristic changes (*see* definition *above*).

Treatment
1. Make a firm diagnosis.
2. Tell the patient—also the prognosis, and the treatment plan.
3. Initiate regular anti-inflammatory therapy to control the symptoms—start with safer drugs like propionic acid derivatives. Try them all if necessary to find the best for each patient.
4. Supplement with simple analgesics on demand, indomethacin at night for morning stiffness, intra-articular steroids for troublesome joints.
5. Review domestic and work situation. Take steps to *preserve* all aspects of the patients' way of life.
6. Rest and joint protection. Period of rest in hospital may be useful in the early stages in acute cases. Splints to rest active joints and prevent deformity (e.g. flexion deformity of knees). Avoid undue stresses and strains.
7. Suppression of disease activity.
   a. *Penicillamine:* 250 mg. daily for the first 2–4 weeks, increasing by 250 mg. daily every 2–4 weeks. Usual maintenance dose is between 500 mg. and 1 g. daily, occasionally up to 2 g. Check W.B.C., platelets, and urine protein at least monthly. Side effects common. For loss of taste or nausea carry on regardless. For rash, vomiting, or thrombocytopenia, stop and restart 250 mg. daily when normal. Proteinuria occurs after 4 months or more; stop if it exceeds 5 g. daily or patient becomes nephrotic.
   b. *Gold* (Myocrisin) 10, 20, 30, 40 mg. I.M. at weekly intervals, then 50 mg. weekly up to 1 g., then maintenance dose of 50 mg. fortnightly, if results good. Check white count and platelets fortnightly, and urine for protein before each injection.
   c. *Immunosuppressive drugs*: azathioprine (50 mg. t.d.s.), chlorambucil (5–10 mg. daily), cyclophosphamide (50–100 mg. daily) reserved for severe or life-threatening disease.
   d. *Hydroxychloroquine*: 200 mg. t.d.s.—mild but sometimes useful; 6-monthly eye tests essential.
8. Continued supervision and management of complications.

Carpal tunnel syndrome: local steroid injection; surgery if this fails.
Ruptured extensor tendons of hand: repair, débridement, and excision of ulnar head.
Atlanto-axial subluxation: no treatment required; caution if anaesthetic needed; spinal fusion only for definite evidence of cord compression.
Baker's cyst, calf cyst, or joint rupture: rest, intra-articular steroids and if symptoms are particularly troublesome, synovectomy.
Foot deformities, corns, etc.: seamless shoes.
Painful metatarsal heads: metatarsal bar insoles; excision if this fails.
For advanced painful disease in any joint consider surgery—Hip: replacement. Knee: double osteotomy or replacement. Ankle: fusion. Wrist: excision of ulnar head.
Felty's Syndrome: avoid steroids; splenectomy may help but benefit often transient; drugs like penicillamine to control the disease.
Sjogren's Syndrome: hypromellose eye drops.
Anaemia: avoid haematinics unless there is clear evidence of deficiency; commonest cause is active disease and best solution is to control it. Some cases due to drugs: stop them.

RHEUMATOID ARTHRITIS (*continued*)

REFERENCES

[1] SHORT, C. L., and others (1957), *Rheumatoid Arthritis*. Boston: Harvard University Press.

[2] ROPES, M. W., and others (1959), *Annals of the Rheumatic Diseases*, **18**, 49.

[3] DIXON, A. St. J. (1969), *Proceedings of the Royal Society of Medicine*, **63**, 677.

[4] HART, F. D. (1969), *British Medical Journal*, **3**, 131.

[5] HART, F. D. (1970), *British Medical Journal*, **2**, 747.

[6] BREWERTON, D. A. (1969), *British Journal of Radiology*, **42**, 487.

[7] BLOCH, K. J., and others (1965), *Medicine*, **44**, 187.

[8] SCADDING, J. G. (1969), *Proceedings of the Royal Society of Medicine*, **62**, 227.

[9] BARNES, C. G., and others (1971), *Annals of the Rheumatic Diseases*, **30**, 359.

[10] KELLGREN, J. H., and others (1958), *British Medical Journal*, **1**, 1193.

[11] JAFFE, I. A. (1970), *Arthritis and Rheumatism*, **13**, 436.

[12] COOPERATING CLINICS (1970), *New England Journal of Medicine*, **283**, 883.

RUBELLA

A common epidemic virus exanthem, which affects children predominantly. After an incubation period of 14–18 days, there is a mild prodromal illness, and on the first or second day a generalized maculopapular rash appears. Complete recovery follows within a week.

Arthritis also occurs after rubella vaccination,[3] particularly with certain strains. It begins between 2 and 4 weeks after vaccination and varies in severity from a mild arthralgia to polyarthritis; joint involvement is similar to that of rubella arthritis with the small joints of the hands prominently affected, usually bilateral and symmetrical. Arthritis commonly lasts a few days but occasionally weeks.

Joint pain following rubella vaccination may also be due to radiculoneuritis affecting either the arm or the leg. In the arm syndrome, patients wake with distressing pain and paraesthesiae in the hands and fingers which last up to 1 hour. In the leg syndrome there is pain behind the knees, most pronounced on waking in the mornings. Characteristically the knees cannot be straightened. Both syndromes begin between 2 and 10 weeks after vaccination and last usually for days, sometimes weeks.

Incidence

Arthritis occurs in 15 per cent of adults; rare in children. Usually synchronous with rash, but may start a few days before or after. M. = F.

Joints affected

M.C.P. or P.I.P. joints in 85 per cent. Often knees, wrists, ankles, elbows. Usually bilateral and symmetrical. Rarely monarticular.

Symptoms

Acute onset of pain and stiffness. Morning stiffness common.

Signs

Swelling, erythema, tenderness.

Course

Complete resolution without sequelae within a few months.

Associations

1. Maculopapular rash.
2. Suboccipital lymphadenopathy.
3. Fever and muscle pains.

XR

Normal.

Laboratory

ESR raised. Leucopenia with relative lymphocytosis. Occasional transient positive latex test. Rubella antibodies demonstrable. Synovial fluid: inflammatory. W.B.C. up to $20,000 \times 10^9$/dl. mostly mononuclears.

Treatment

Analgesic and anti-inflammatory drugs.

Variant

Arthritis also occurs after rubella vaccination (*see above*).

REFERENCES

[1] CHAMBERS, R. J., and BYWATERS, E. G. L. (1963), *Annals of the Rheumatic Diseases*, **22**, 263.

[2] FRY, J., and others (1962), *British Medical Journal*, **2**, 833.

[3] LERMAN, S. J., and others (1971), *Annals of Internal Medicine*, **74**, 67.

[4] KILROY, A. W., and others (1970), *Journal of the American Medical Association*, **214**, 2287.

SACRO-ILIAC STRAIN

A common condition particularly found in nurses and other occupations where heavy lifting is required. There is pain in one or both sacro-iliac joints which may radiate down the back of the thigh to the knee, aggravated by movement and relieved by rest. Tenderness over the joint is sometimes found. The first episode is occasionally acute, severe, and disabling but tends to get better within a few weeks; recurrence is common and the condition may become chronic though most cases are symptom-free within a few years. E.S.R. and XR of the sacro-iliac joints are normal. Treatment: Rest and phenylbutazone or indomethacin in the acute stage; later simple analgesics as required. Change of occupation may be desirable.

SALMONELLA ARTHRITIS

Arthritis due to direct infection of a joint with *Salmonella*. The manifestations of *Salmonella* infections vary with the causative organism. *S. typhi* causes a severe febrile illness with a mortality of about 5 per cent. Enteric fever (paratyphoid) is a milder febrile illness with diarrhoea; the remainder cause 'food poisoning', a predominantly gastro-intestinal illness.

Incidence
M. = F.
Any age but usually children (80 per cent).
Arthritis occurs in 0·25 per cent of all cases of *Salmonella* infection and 2·5 per cent of cases of infection with *S. choleraesuis*.

Joints affected
Knee commonest (60 per cent).
Shoulder (40 per cent); hip (15 per cent).
Rarely ankle, elbow, sacro-iliac joint, or temporomandibular joint.
One to four joints, monarticular in 60 per cent.
Usually asymmetrical.

Symptoms
Sudden onset of pain and swelling.

Signs
Joint is swollen with effusion, tenderness, and limitation of movement.
Erythema and warmth occasionally.
Periarticular oedema rare.
Fever usual.

Course
Untreated arthritis becomes chronic.
Treated cases recover completely without sequelae within 3 months.

Associations
1. Diarrhoea often absent.
2. Splenomegaly in 30 per cent.

XR
Usually normal.
Porosis, bone destruction, and osteomyelitis are late features.

Laboratory
Mild leucocytosis in 75 per cent.
Synovial fluid: purulent; W.B.C. 10–100,000 $\times 10^9$/dl.; predominantly neutrophils. Culture usually positive.
Organism may be cultured from stools and sometimes blood.
Positive agglutination test; rising titre.

Treatment
1. Chloramphenicol.
2. Rest in acute stage.
3. Daily aspiration until effusion disappears.

Variants
1. Salmonella osteomyelitis is particularly common in patients with sickle-cell disease.[2]
2. Post-salmonella arthritis (*see* p. 91).
3. Typhoid fever (*see* p. 145).

REFERENCES

[1] DAVID, J. R., and BLACK, R. L. (1960), *Medicine*, **39**, 385.

[2] HOOK, E. W. (1961), *Bulletin of the New York Academy of Medicine*, **37**, 499.

SARCOIDOSIS

A condition of unknown aetiology characterized pathologically by granulomatous inflammation, particularly affecting lymph-nodes, spleen, liver, and lungs. Two types of arthritis occur.

1. *Early Acute Transient Type*: a polyarthritis of the type which is associated with erythema nodosum. This occurs in 20 per cent of cases of sarcoidosis at or soon after the onset of the disease and is usually (in 70 per cent of cases) but not always associated with erythema nodosum. Arthritis and erythema nodosum are more common in the Irish, Puerto Ricans, and Swedish. Arthritis is usually symmetrical affecting the knees and ankles particularly and is fully described on p. 30. The most useful diagnostic test is a chest X-ray, which shows hilar lymphadenopathy in 80 per cent.

2. *Chronic Persistent Type*: a polyarthritis associated with chronic sarcoidosis.

Incidence
F. 3 : 1.
Age 15–50, peak 20–30.
Affects 10 per cent of patients with sarcoidosis.
Onset usually in the first year of the disease.

Joints affected
Polyarticular.
Knees and ankles commonly affected.
Often elbows, wrists, shoulders, M.C.P. and P.I.P. joints of hands. Occasionally feet, hips, and spine.
Rarely affects the big toe, resembling gout.
Usually symmetrical (80 per cent).

Symptoms
Sudden or gradual onset of pain and swelling.
Morning stiffness.

Signs
Red, warm, swollen joint with effusion in the acute stage.
Limitation of movement.
Fever occasionally.

Course
Chronic; lasts for years with relapses and remissions but usually subsides eventually.
Deformities are rare and slight.

Associations
1. Other manifestations of chronic sarcoidosis; peripheral lymphadenopathy (80 per cent), cutaneous sarcoid (50 per cent), iritis (30 per cent), and involvement of other organs. Changes on CXR common (*see below*).
2. Rarely tenosynovitis or carpal tunnel syndrome.

XR
Joints usually normal. Cystic changes are occasionally seen in hands or feet.
CXR shows hilar lymphadenopathy (75 per cent) and/or pulmonary infiltration (50 per cent).

Laboratory
Raised E.S.R. in active phase.
Latex test positive in 10 per cent.
Hypergammaglobulinaemia in 60 per cent.
Hypercalcaemia in 10 per cent.
Hyperuricaemia in 10 per cent.
Mantoux test negative in 70 per cent.
Kveim test positive in 70 per cent.
Biopsy of synovium or other affected tissues (lymph-nodes, skin, or liver) shows granulomata and inflammatory changes.
Synovial fluid: inflammatory with neutrophil leucocytosis.

Treatment
Anti-inflammatory and analgesic drugs.
Steroids only for severe cases resistant to other therapy or for other indications, e.g., iritis and hypercalcaemia.

REFERENCE

GUMPEL, J. M., and others (1967), *Annals of the Rheumatic Diseases*, **26**, 194.

SCARLET FEVER

Infection with certain strains of *Streptococcus*. The condition is at present rare and mild; its former reputation was due to the association of acute nephritis and rheumatic fever. After an incubation period of 2–6 days, the patient (usually a child) develops a sore throat, fever, headache and malaise. On the second day, a punctate erythema appears on the face, spreading to the trunk and limbs, and fading with some peeling within a week.

Joint manifestations are of four types:

1. Arthralgia is often noted in the early febrile illness.

2. A transient arthritis may occur particularly between the fifth and seventh days in older children and adults, and is commoner in females. The upper limb is commonly involved, particularly the wrists and M.C.P. joints, which are painful and swollen. Complete recovery follows within a few days.

3. Septic arthritis (*see* p. 123) may complicate septicaemia.

4. Rheumatic fever (*see* p. 113) occurs 2–3 weeks after onset.

The diagnosis is usually made on the clinical features; a throat swab confirms the presence of streptococci. Treatment: Penicillin.

REFERENCE

Christie, A. B. (1955), *Rheumatism*, **11**, 68.

SCLERODERMA

A condition characterized by inflammation of subcutaneous connective tissue (oedema and lymphocytic infiltration in the early stages) followed by progressive fibrosis leading to secondary atrophy of the skin, subcutaneous fat, sweat-glands, and hair follicles. This is accompanied by arteritis of the skin vessels. A similar fibrotic process may occur in other organs, particularly the oesophagus. Apart from the arthritis described below, avascular necrosis of the femoral head and neuropathic joints have been rarely described.

Incidence

F. 3 : 1.
Peak age 20–50.
Joints affected in most cases, early in the course of the disease.

Joints affected

Fingers commonest.
Any other joint may be affected.
Often symmetrical.
Resembles rheumatoid arthritis in early stages.

Symptoms

Pain, swelling, and stiffness.
Morning stiffness.

Signs

Joints may be swollen, tender, and warm in early stages; later signs of inflammation disappear.
Flexion deformities of fingers common.

Course

Arthritis usually abates within the first year and is seldom a problem.
Five-year survival 75 per cent; 10 years 50 per cent.
Worse prognosis with onset over 40, renal, pulmonary, or cardiac involvement and skin changes affecting the trunk.

Associations

A. *Skin Changes*
1. Early oedema.
2. Eventually the skin is hard, smooth, shiny, and bound down to underlying structures.
3. Telangiectasis (75 per cent) in affected areas.
4. Pigmentation (50 per cent)—may resemble Addison's disease.
5. Ulceration of finger-tips, knuckles, or lower legs (40 per cent).
6. Calcinosis (10 per cent).

B. *Visceral Changes*
1. Raynaud's phenomenon (common).
2. Dysphagia (65 per cent); rarely malabsorption or hepatic fibrosis.
3. Tendinitis (35 per cent) causes crepitus, and contractures.
4. Obliterative endarteritis of renal vessels causes renal failure in 20 per cent with proteinuria and malignant hypertension.
5. Sjögren's syndrome (6 per cent).
6. Fibrosing alveolitis (rare).
7. Interstitial myocardial fibrosis rarely causes arrhythmia or conduction defects. Pericarditis, valve lesions, and cardiomyopathy very rare.
8. Features of other connective-tissue disorders—*see* Mixed Connective-tissue Disease. (p. 75).

XR

1. Resorption of tufts of distal phalanges.
2. Subcutaneous calcification.
3. Joint narrowing.
4. Periarticular osteoporosis.
   Barium swallow useful to show oesophageal changes.

Laboratory

E.S.R. raised (50 per cent).
Positive latex test (30 per cent).
Positive A.N.F. (80 per cent).
L.E. cells (10 per cent).

Treatment

Analgesic and anti-inflammatory drugs.
Steroids and penicillamine have no beneficial effect on skin changes.

REFERENCES

RODNAN, G. P. (1962), *Annals of Internal Medicine*, 56, 422.

KARTEN, I. (1970), *Arthritis and Rheumatism*, 12, 636.

SCURVY

Vitamin-C deficiency in infants is manifest predominantly as a disease of bone and joints[1]. It used to occur in babies fed on artificial milk, but has been almost eliminated by the use of regular vitamin supplements. Clinically it may resemble Still's disease (but occurs at an earlier age), or the arthritis of acute leukaemia. Scurvy in adults also causes arthritis. It may be dietary and also occurs in South African Bantu who drink large amounts of iron-containing beer.[2] This condition occurs in middle-aged men and is associated with osteoporosis, avascular necrosis of the hip and sometimes cirrhosis and other manifestations of haemochromatosis.

Incidence

M. = F.
Infantile type age 6–18 months.

Joints affected .

Usually hips and knees.
Upper limbs affected later and less severely: wrists and shoulders.
Bilateral but asymmetrical.

Symptoms

Infants:
Sudden or gradual onset of fretfulness with pain, and screaming on moving lower limbs.
Adults:
Aching bones and joints.
Swollen joints.

Signs

1. Painful limitation of movement. The infant prefers to lie still with the hips in a flexed everted position.
2. Extreme tenderness of bone ends.
3. Swelling of the knees; effusion and sometimes crepitus. Often slight fever.

Course

Chronic.
Rapid response to vitamin C.

Associations

1. Haemorrhage. Perifollicular haemorrhages over upper thighs and abdomen; petechiae; easy bruising; haematuria; retro-orbital haemorrhage may cause proptosis.
2. Swollen bleeding gums.
3. Pallor.

XR

Changes best seen in femur and tibia of infants.
1. Porosis; wide medullary spaces with loss of trabeculation; narrow cortex.
2. Widening of the ends of long bones.
3. Subperiosteal haemorrhages, later calcified.
4. A line of sclerosis is seen at the ends of metaphyses and in a ring around the epiphyses.
5. Metaphyseal spurs.
6. Fragmentation of bone ends or fractures.
7. Costal beading.

Laboratory

Anaemia.
Leucocytosis.
Leucocyte ascorbic acid level low.
Ascorbic acid saturation test.
Synovial fluid: blood-stained.

Treatment

1. Ascorbic acid 100 mg. daily.
2. Careful handling until healing occurs.

REFERENCES

[1] BARLOW, T. (1894), *Lancet*, **2**, 1075.

[2] SEFTEL, H. C., and others (1966), *British Medical Journal*, **1**, 642.

SEPTIC ARTHRITIS

Infection of a joint with pyogenic bacteria. The commonest organism is *Staphylococcus aureus* (50 per cent); *Streptococcus pyogenes*, *Str. faecalis*, *Str. viridans*, *Pneumococcus*, *E. coli*, *Haemophilus influenzae*, *Proteus*, *Pseudomonas aeruginosa*, *Klebsiella*, *Aerobacter*, *Vibrio fetus*, and *Serratia* may cause an identical clinical picture. Infection with anaerobic organisms is considered separately (*see* p. 6). Other organisms which cause arthritis are listed in the classification (*see* p. iii).

Incidence

M. 2 : 1.
Any age but particularly childhood and old age.
Rare complication of infection elsewhere; predisposing factors present in 70 per cent, e.g.,
1. Diabetes mellitus.
2. Rheumatoid arthritis.
3. Joint puncture or surgery.
4. Steroid therapy.
5. Debilitating diseases.

Joints affected

Knee commonest (50 per cent).
Occasionally hip, shoulder, elbow, wrist, sternoclavicular joint, or ankle.
Others rare.
90 per cent monarticular.

Symptoms

Rapid onset of severe pain and swelling occasionally preceded by generalized arthralgia.

Signs

Swelling with effusion, tenderness, warmth, and painful limitation of movement.
Joint often red.
Periarticular oedema occasionally.
Fever usual.

Course

Untreated, proceeds rapidly to joint destruction. Complications:
1. Osteomyelitis.
2. Sinus formation.
3. Ankylosis.
4. Dislocation of the hip.

XR

Normal at first.
1. Osteoporosis appears after about 2 weeks.
2. Destructive changes rare and late.

Laboratory

Leucocytosis (90 per cent).
Synovial fluid: purulent; W.B.C. up to $200,000 \times 10^9/dl.$; 90 per cent neutrophils.
Gram stain shows organisms in 50 per cent.
Culture usually positive (85 per cent); if negative, repeat and ask for anaerobic culture.
Blood-culture often positive.

Treatment

1. Antibiotics (oral or I.M.).
2. Rest in acute stage. Sometimes splints and traction.
3. Daily aspiration; open drainage and débridement indicated for (*a*) failure to resolve, (*b*) joints inaccessible to aspiration, e.g., hip.
4. Intra-articular antibiotics usually unnecessary except to give toxic antibiotics such as polymyxin. Repeated intra-articular injection of large doses of antibiotics leads to 'post-infectious synovitis' with return of pain, warmth, tenderness, and effusion. Synovial fluid is sterile with high W.B.C. Treat with rest.
5. Physiotherapy required later to restore full range of movement and muscle power.

REFERENCES

ARGEN, R. J., and others (1966), *Archives of Internal Medicine*, **117**, 661.
CHARTIER, Y., and others (1959), *Annals of Internal Medicine*, **50**, 1462.
HEBERLING, J. A. (1941), *Journal of Bone and Joint Surgery*, **23**, 917.
WARD, J., and others (1960), *Arthritis and Rheumatism*, **3**, 522.

SEPTIC FOCUS SYNDROME

A very rare condition in which arthralgia, sometimes with joint swelling, is associated with a focus of infection usually in the teeth, tonsils, or pelvis. Drainage or removal of the septic focus is followed by disappearance of the joint pain. One or many joints may be affected, and there is no particular pattern.

REFERENCE

HART, F. D. (1970), *Annals of Physical Medicine*, **10**, 257.

SERUM SICKNESS

An immune complex-mediated systemic reaction to injections of foreign protein or drugs. It begins 7–14 days after exposure or earlier (after 1–4 days) if there has been previous sensitization. There is fever, often an urticarial rash, and a few days later pain and swelling of joints. Knees, ankles and wrists are most commonly affected in a bilateral symmetrical distribution. Joints are tender and swollen with effusions. There may be lymphadenopathy, erythematous rashes or purpura. XR normal. Joint fluid: inflammatory; WBC up to $20,000 \times 10^9$/dl., mainly polymorphs. Serum complement: low. WBC and ESR: normal or raised.

SEVER'S DISEASE

A condition resembling tennis elbow, but occurring at the attachment of the posterior apophysis of the calcaneus to the bone. It affects children aged 8–13 and presents with pain in the heel and local tenderness. Treatment: Rest; local injection of prednisolone.

SHOULDER–HAND SYNDROME

Painful disability of the shoulder, preceding, accompanying, or following pain, swelling, and vasomotor changes in the hand and fingers. This may be: (1) *idiopathic* (25 per cent), or may occur (2) after *myocardial infarction* (20 per cent). (3) In association with *cervical spondylosis* (20 per cent). (4) After *trauma* (10 per cent). (5) After *hemiplegia* (5 per cent). (6) With *drugs*, phenobarbitone,[2] isoniazid or ethionamide,[3] and (7) with *malignancy* either pulmonary (Pancoast syndrome) or cerebral; any type of arthritis of the shoulder; herpes zoster.

Incidence
F. 3 : 2.
Age 30+, usually 50–70.
Affects 1 per cent of cases of myocardial infarction (but up to 20 per cent if completely immobilized); starts 1 week to 6 months after infarct.

Joints affected
Shoulder, wrist, and hand.
25 per cent bilateral.
Elbow rare (5 per cent).

Symptoms
Pain in shoulder usually preceding diffuse pain in hand by a few weeks.
Hand affected first in 10 per cent.
Weakness of limb.
No morning stiffness.

Signs
Shoulder: painful limitation of movement; tenderness.
Hand: diffuse pitting oedema (often marked over dorsum) and tenderness.
Skin: warm, moist, shiny, and hyperaesthetic.

Course
Hand swelling either resolves completely in 1–6 months or rarely induration and atrophy of skin appear with flexion contractures of fingers.
Permanent restriction of shoulder movement may result but more often the condition subsides after 1 or 2 years.
Recurrence rare.

XR
Patchy osteoporosis of hand appears after weeks or months.

Laboratory
E.S.R. normal in 80 per cent.
W.B.C. normal.
Thermography: diffusely raised temperature (not confined to joints as in rheumatoid arthritis).

Treatment
1. Analgesic/anti-inflammatory drugs.
2. Exercises to maintain mobility. Local heat or cold may help.
3. ACTH or steroids.
4. Stellate ganglion block.
5. Local steroid injection of tender areas.

Prophylaxis: avoid immobility after myocardial infarction, stroke, or trauma.

REFERENCES

[1] STEINBROCKER, O., and ARGYROS, T. G. (1958), *Medical Clinics of North America*, **42**, 1533.
[2] VAN DER KORST, J. K., and others (1966), *Annals of the Rheumatic Diseases*, **25**, 553.
[3] GOOD, A. E., and others (1965), *Annals of Internal Medicine*, **63**, 800.

SICKLE-CELL DISEASE

A condition inherited as an autosomal intermediate, in which haemoglobin A is replaced by haemoglobin S. Heterozygotes are not anaemic and do not have arthritis. Homozygotes are severely anaemic and have thrombotic crises which commonly cause arthritis as a result of local bone infarcts. The condition is found in Negroes particularly in tropical Africa and less commonly in the U.S.A., around the Mediterranean, the Middle East, and India. Similar thrombotic crises with arthritis occur in haemoglobin sickle-cell disease and sickle-cell thalassaemia.

Incidence

M. = F.
Onset usually in the first 10 years of life.
90 per cent have episodes of arthritis at some time; arthritis is a prominent feature of 50 per cent of crises.

Joints affected

Polyarticular.
Hands and feet common; may affect any other joints. Bilateral and symmetrical. Often migratory.

Symptoms

Sudden onset of severe joint pains or backache. Crises may be precipitated by infection. Bone pain common.

Signs

Often none.
Affected joints are occasionally swollen, red, warm, or tender, sometimes with effusion. Fever common in crises.

Course

Joint pain subsides spontaneously within a few days but may recur with subsequent crises.
Life span is considerably reduced and death in childhood is common.

Associations

1. Chronic anaemia and intermittent jaundice.
2. Crises may also cause abdominal pain (simulating intra-abdominal catastrophe), pulmonary or cerebral infarction.
3. Chronic leg ulcers (40 per cent).
4. Slight splenomegaly in young children, disappearing later; hepatomegaly.
5. Cholelithiasis (30 per cent).

XR

1. Areas of porosis or sclerosis of bone (representing infarcts).
2. Dactylitis (periosteal proliferation affecting shafts of metatarsals, metacarpals, or phalanges sometimes with cystic changes).
3. Evidence of bone-marrow hyperplasia (wide medulla, thin cortex, porosis; hair-on-end appearance of skull).
4. Avascular necrosis.
5. Look for salmonella osteomyelitis (destruction of bone with periosteal proliferation; usually multiple sites).

Laboratory

In vitro sickling tests and haemoglobin electrophoresis confirm the diagnosis. Haemoglobin about 50 per cent; cells hypochromic.
Reticulocytosis.
Bilirubin slightly raised.
Leucocytosis in crises.

Treatment

1. Analgesics in crisis.
2. Intravenous bicarbonate infusion may help.
3. Avoid anoxia, hypotension, tourniquets, and blood transfusion.

Variant

Avascular necrosis occurs in 10 per cent usually affecting the head of the femur. Rarely affects knee, shoulder, or vertebrae.

REFERENCES

CARROLL, D. S. (1957), *Southern Medical Journal*, **50**, 1486.
LAMBOTTE, C. (1962), *American Journal of Diseases of Children*, **104**, 200.
SMITH, E. W., and CONLEY, C. L. (1954), *Bulletin of the Johns Hopkins Hospital*, **94**, 289.

SMALLPOX (Variola)

An uncommon virus infection. After an incubation period of 12 days, there is a febrile toxaemic illness, followed 2 days later by a rash which is in turn macular, papular, vesicular, and pustular, affecting particularly the extremities. Complications are common and potentially fatal. Arthritis is secondary to infection of adjacent bone (Osteomyelitis variolosa).

Incidence

M. = F.
Arthritis in 5 per cent under age 10: very rare over this age.
Usually unvaccinated.
Onset 1–4 weeks after appearance of rash.

Joints affected

Elbows commonest (80 per cent); also wrists or small joints of hands (20 per cent), ankles or feet (10 per cent), knees (10 per cent), and shoulders (10 per cent).
Commonly bilateral and symmetrical.

Symptoms

Insidious onset of joint swelling and limitation of movement.
Pain often slight or absent at onset, but severe later.

Signs

Periarticular swelling extending into the soft tissues above and below the joint.
Effusion occasionally present.
Limitation of movement.
Late features: abnormal mobility, crepitus and discharging sinuses. Fever common.

Course

Arthritis settles within 3 months but some residual disability is common, e.g., limitation of motion or deformity; occasionally ankylosis, destructive changes resembling a neuropathic joint, or limb shortening.

Associations

Desquamating skin lesions.

XR

1. Metaphyseal osteoporosis.
2. Destructive changes in the metaphysis with irregularity of joint surface and new bone formation along the shaft of the bone.
3. Detachment or displacement of the epiphysis.

Laboratory

Leucocytosis and raised E.S.R.
Synovial fluid: leucocytosis; elementary bodies may be seen; culture for secondary bacterial infection.

Treatment

1. Immobilize affected joints in plaster in acute stage.
2. Analgesics.

REFERENCE

COCKSHOTT, P., and McGREGOR, M. (1958), *Quarterly Journal of Medicine*, 27, 369.

SUDECK'S ATROPHY

A condition of unknown aetiology in which painful swelling of a joint with porosis of bone follows local trauma. The condition is distinguished from traumatic arthritis because the clinical manifestations are delayed in onset and disproportionately prolonged. A very similar condition occurs in the absence of trauma and is described as Transient Painful Osteoporosis (p. 140).

Predisposing Factors

1. Trauma in 70 per cent—injury may be minor but particularly common after fractures.
2. Surgery in 25 per cent.
3. Remainder follow burns or other injuries.

Incidence

M. 3 : 2.
Any age, peak 30–60.
Usually begins within days or weeks of trauma—60 per cent within the first month, 30 per cent up to 6 months and 10 per cent later.

Joints affected

Monarticular. Ankle commonest (85 per cent), sometimes wrist (15 per cent).

Symptoms

1. Progressively increasing severe burning aching pain.
2. Local hyperaesthesia or less often paraesthesia.

SUDECK'S ATROPHY (*continued*)

3. Swelling.
4. Stiffness.
5. Pain on weight-bearing or movement; relief with rest.
6. Sweating.

Signs
1. Tenderness of the affected joint and surrounding areas. Hyperaesthesia of surrounding skin.
2. Diffuse soft-tissue swelling around the joint.
3. Erythema of overlying skin sometimes. Skin is typically smooth and glossy— it may be warmer or cooler than normal and there is sometimes increased sweating.
4. Painful restriction of movement.
5. Muscle wasting.

Course
The condition usually resolves spontaneously over the course of a few months.

Permanent stiffness with atrophy of skin and muscle may result after prolonged immobilization.

XR
Patchy osteoporosis.

Laboratory
E.S.R. may be raised but no specific findings. Bone biopsy: atrophy.

Treatment
1. Anti-inflammatory drugs to relieve pain.
2. Ankle physiotherapy to maintain mobility.
If severe symptoms persist try:
3. Immobilization in plaster (walking plaster for lower limb).
If still troublesome:
4. Consider stellate ganglion block—if this is not effective, sympathectomy may work but such extreme measures are seldom required.

REFERENCE

KLEINERT, H. E., and others (1972), *Journal of Bone and Joint Surgery*, **54A**, 899.

SWEET'S SYNDROME (Acute Febrile Neutrophilic Dermatosis)

A disease characterized by fever, leucocytosis, and raised tender plaques or nodules on the skin of the face, neck and limbs, biopsy of which show dense dermal infiltration with neutrophils.

Incidence
Rare.
Middle-aged women most often affected.
Arthritis in 20 per cent, at the time of development of the fever and skin lesions.

Joints affected
Small joints of hands, wrists, elbows, ankles, knees. Bilateral and symmetrical.

Symptoms
Acute onset of pain and swelling.

Signs
Warmth, swelling and tenderness. Sometimes small effusions.

Course
Arthritis is transient lasting days or weeks, no sequelae. Rash lasts for weeks or months.

About one-third of cases have recurrence.
Rapid and complete response to steroids.

Associations
1. Skin lesions: raised well-defined tender dull red or purple plaques, 0·5–4 cm. in diameter, developing asymmetrically on the face and limbs, appearing over 2–3 weeks, becoming confluent and healing without scarring within a few months. Lesions on the lower limb resemble erythema nodosum. Histology: infiltration with neutrophils.
2. Fatigue, malaise and fever in the first week of the illness. Fever may precede rash by up to 3 weeks.
3. Occasionally episcleritis or glomerulitis.

XR
Normal.

SWEET'S SYNDROME (Acute Febrile Neutrophilic Dermatosis) (*continued*)

Laboratory
W.B.C.: neutrophil leucocytosis.
Raised E.S.R.
Latex test and A.N.F. negative.
Synovial fluid: mildy inflammatory. Mainly mononuclear cells.

Treatment
Symptomatic therapy often sufficient—steroids if not.

REFERENCES

KRANSER, R. E., and SCHUMACHER, M. R. (1975), *Arthritis and Rheumatism*, **18**, 35.

SWEET, R. D. (1964), *British Journal of Dermatology*, **76**, 349.

SYNOVIOMA (Synovial Sarcoma)

A rare highly malignant tumour which arises in synovial membrane or in the soft tissues around the joint (tendons, tendon sheaths, and bursae). Histologically there are two components, spindle cells (typical of fibrosarcoma), and epithelioid cells.

Incidence
M. = F.
Any age, peak 20–60.

Joints affected
Lower limb 2 : 1.
Knee and thigh are commonest sites; any other joint may be affected.
Monarticular.

Symptoms
1. Swelling.
2. Pain in 60 per cent.
Symptoms begin insidiously, often several years before the patient presents, and are mild.

Signs
Soft-tissue swelling.
Tenderness occasionally.

Course
Early metastases to local lymph-nodes or lung are common, and may appear many years after excision of the primary.
Prognosis is poor; 10 per cent survive 10 years.

XR
1. Soft-tissue mass. Rarely shows spotty calcification.
2. Later erosion of adjacent bone.
Chest X-ray for metastases.

Laboratory
Unhelpful.

Treatment
Radical surgery: wide excision or amputation depending on position.
Recurrence is very common after local excision.
The tumour is not particularly radiosensitive.

Variants
A similar clinical picture may be produced by other soft-tissue sarcomata.

REFERENCES

CADMAN, N. L., and others (1965), *Cancer*, **18**, 613.
HAMPOLE, M. K., and JACKSON, B. A. (1968), *Canadian Medical Association Journal*, **99**, 1025.

TILLOTSON, J. F., and others (1951), *Journal of Bone and Joint Surgery*, **33A**, 459.

SYPHILIS

Venereal infection with *Treponema pallidum*, causing at first a genital chancre (primary syphilis) followed a few weeks later by a febrile illness (secondary syphilis), and many years later by gummata, cardiovascular or neurological disorders (tertiary syphilis). Congenital syphilis affects the children of syphilitic mothers. All types are a little commoner in men (M. 3 : 2), and particularly affect young adults. The disease has become rare.

Arthritis is of seven types:

1. *Clutton's Joints* (*see* p. 20), bilateral hydrarthrosis of the knee in congenital syphilis.
2. *Neuropathic Joint* (*see* p. 83) in tertiary syphilis, is a complication of tabes dorsalis.
3. *Arthralgia* is a common feature of secondary syphilis, associated with fever and a rash, and responding rapidly to penicillin.
4. *Synovitis*, resembling Clutton's joints, may occur either with late secondary or early tertiary syphilis.

Joints affected
Knees commonest; one often precedes the other.
Eventually bilateral but asymmetrical.
Occasionally elbows or ankles.

Symptoms
Swelling.
Pain mild or absent.

Signs
Effusion.
Joints are not usually red, warm, or tender.

Course
Variable duration (up to 1 year) but eventually complete resolution without residua.

XR
Normal.

Laboratory
W.R. positive.
Synovial fluid: inflammatory with polymorph leucocytosis.

Treatment
Penicillin should be given but may have little or no effect on arthritis.

5. *Gummatous Arthritis* is a rare feature of tertiary, or late congenital syphilis, and is due to gumma formation either in the joint or in adjacent bone.

Joints affected
Monarticular.
Knee commonest.
Sometimes ankle, wrist, elbow, shoulder, or hip.
Small joints rare.

Symptoms
Joint swelling.
Pain mild or absent.

Signs
Effusion without warmth or erythema of overlying skin.
Sometimes tenderness and 'lumpy swelling'.

Course
Chronic but only slowly progressive.
Ankylosis or discharging sinuses may develop eventually in untreated cases.
Osteoarthritis may be a complication, particularly in hip or knee.

XR
Localized bone destruction.
Periosteal reaction.
Large osteophytes.

Laboratory
W.R. usually positive.

Treatment
Pencillin produces rapid resolution.
Rest required in acute stage.

SYPHILIS (*continued*)

6. *Spondylitis* is also rare and occurs in late secondary, tertiary, or congenital syphilis.

Joints affected

Cervical spine (70 per cent), dorsal (15 per cent), lumbar (15 per cent).
Localized to one to five vertebrae.

Symptoms

Pain and stiffness.

Signs

Painful limitation of movement.
Local tenderness.

Course

Chronic and slowly progressive.
May lead to ankylosis of the affected segment of the spine.
Cord compression rare.

XR

Destruction of vertebral body with surrounding sclerosis and new bone foundation.
Later calcification of anterior and lateral ligament with large osteophytes.

Laboratory

Positive W.R. in 80 per cent.

Treatment

Penicillin is rapidly effective.
Immobilization in a collar or plaster cast may be required while healing takes place.

7. *Non-articular Causes* of joint pain include *periostitis*, said to be the commonest skeletal lesion of late syphilis. Commonest sites are the tibia and shoulder girdle; XR shows a well-defined area of subperiosteal rarefaction. Penicillin produces rapid resolution.

Osteochondritis occurs in congenital syphilis in the first 3 months of life. The upper limbs are particularly affected and X-rays are diagnostic. Complete resolution follows early treatment with penicillin, but deformities may result if treatment is delayed. *Bursitis* and tendon *nodules* are rare.

REFERENCES

FREEDMAN, E., and MESCHAN, I. (1943), *American Journal of Roentgenology*, **49**, 756.
McEWEN, C., and THOMAS, E. W. (1938), *Medical Clinics of North America*, **22**, 1275.

STOKES, J. H., and others (1944), *Modern Clinical Syphilology*. Philadelphia: Saunders.

SYSTEMIC LUPUS ERYTHEMATOSUS (S.L.E.)

A condition possibly caused by circulating immune complexes and characterized by the presence of antinuclear factor and other auto-antibodies. The diagnosis is often made on the basis of multi-system involvement. In some cases there are features of other connective-tissue disorders (Mixed Connective-tissue Disease—p. 75). Avascular necrosis (p. 10) has been reported with or without corticosteroid therapy. Drug-induced S.L.E. is described on p. 26.

Incidence

F. 9 : 1.
Any age, peak 20–40.
Commoner in Negroes in U.S.A.
Joint pain in 90 per cent of cases (presenting feature in 50 per cent).
Arthritis usually occurs at onset but may precede other systemic features by up to 20 years.

Joints affected

Polyarticular, distribution resembling rheumatoid arthritis.
Commonly affects P.I.P. and M.C.P. joints of hands, wrists, knees, ankles, elbows, and shoulders.
Often cervical spine, hips, and temporo-mandibular joints.
Bilateral and symmetrical, occasionally migratory.

Symptoms

Sudden onset of pain and stiffness, which may be precipitated by exposure to sunlight or stress.
Morning stiffness in 50 per cent.

Signs

About 50 per cent have none; most characteristic finding is slight soft-tissue swelling only; signs often disproportionate to symptoms.
Occasionally tenderness, warmth, erythema, or effusion.
Fever common (90 per cent).

Course

70 per cent survive 5 years; 50 per cent 10 years. Prognosis much worse with renal involvement.
Arthritis is often mild and either chronic or episodic. Attacks recur at irregular intervals, months or years apart, and last for days or months. In most cases the arthritis leaves no deformity but about 20 per cent develop either swan-neck deformities or ulnar deviation (resembling Jaccoud's syndrome, *see* p. 60). These can be distinguished from rheumatoid deformities by the absence of erosions on XR; the deformities can often be corrected voluntarily.

XR

Usually normal. Rarely,
1. Erosions.
2. Porosis, joint narrowing, and bone destruction.
3. Avascular necrosis (hip, knee, or shoulder).
4. Atlanto-axial subluxation.

Laboratory

E.S.R. raised (85 per cent).
A.N.F. always positive.
L.E. cells present (80 per cent).
Positive latex test (30 per cent).
Positive W.R. (25 per cent).
Serum complement low and anti-DNA antibodies present in cases with active disease and especially renal involvement.
Mild anaemia common. Neutropenia (65 per cent) or thrombocytopenia (20 per cent).
Haemolytic anaemia with positive Coombs' test (5 per cent).
Hyperglobulinaemia often.
Synovial fluid: non-inflammatory; viscous; W.B.C. less than $10,000 \times 10^9/dl.$, predominantly mononuclear. Complement level often low.
Biopsy of skin or kidney occasionally diagnostic.

Treatment

1. Prednisolone for cases with severe systemic disease; 30–60mg. daily at first (sometimes up to 120 mg. required), reducing slowly to a maintenance dose of about 15 mg. daily.
2. Rest in acute stage.
3. Azathioprine useful for steroid-sparing effect (e.g., in patients developing steroid side-effects).
4. Add cyclophosphamide or chlorambucil in patients with progressive renal disease.
5. Chloroquine for mild cases and skin involvement.
6. Avoid pregnancy in acute stage. Avoid sunlight.
7. Plasmapheresis in the desperate case.

SYSTEMIC LUPUS ERYTHEMATOSUS (S.L.E.) *(continued)*

Associations

Skin (80 per cent): Presenting manifestation in 20 per cent.
1. Cutaneous erythema or maculopapular rash on light-exposed areas of face (butterfly area) and upper trunk. Sensitivity to sunlight in 30 per cent.
2. Vasculitic lesions on the fingers: splinter haemorrhages, nail-fold lesions, Osler's nodes, cutaneous infarcts, gangrene.
3. Purpura and bruises.
4. Urticaria and angioneurotic oedema.
5. Discoid lesions.
6. Alopecia, diffuse or focal 'lupus hair'.
7. Hyperpigmentation either diffuse or localized; localized hypopigmentation.
8. Mucous membrane lesions: petechiae or ulcers. Rarely bullae which may be haemorrhagic, areas of thickened bounddown skin which resemble scleroderma, leg ulcers, livedo reticularis, or nodular panniculitis.

Renal (65 per cent): Presenting manifestation in only 5 per cent but occurs usually in the first few years of the disease. Routine urinalysis or renal function tests often show abnormalities; may lead to progressive renal failure or nephrotic syndrome.

Lungs (50 per cent):
1. Pleurisy usually with effusion (40 per cent).
2. Recurrent pneumonitis: fever, dyspnoea, cyanosis, plate atelectasis on CXR.
3. Unexplained dyspnoea may be due to airways obstruction, diffusion defect, reduced vital capacity, or reduced lung compliance.

Cardiovascular (50 per cent):
1. Pericarditis (30 per cent). Tamponade or constriction uncommon.
2. Hypertension (25 per cent).
3. Murmurs (20 per cent) but many are functional; Libman-Sacks endocarditis (predominantly mitral valve); lone aortic incompetence.
4. Myocarditis secondary to coronary vasculitis. Heart failure unusual except in terminal state.

Nervous System (50 per cent): Mostly central.
1. Disorders of mental function (30 per cent): depression, paranoia, anxiety, confusion, schizophrenia, hallucinations, dementia.
2. Fits (10 per cent).
3. Chorea.
4. Vascular accidents.
5. Encephalomyelitis: coma.
6. Peripheral neuropathy (5 per cent): either symmetrical sensorimotor, mononeuritis multiplex or motor neuropathy resembling Guillain-Barré syndrome but with gradual onset.
7. Cranial nerve lesions causing abnormalities of extraocular movement of pupils. Fundi may show haemorrhages (10 per cent) or cytoid bodies (10 per cent).
Rarely transverse myelitis (paraplegia) or subarachnoid haemorrhage. C.S.F. often normal but may show raised protein or increased cells.

Hepatomegaly (25 per cent) but not jaundice. Biopsy unhelpful.

Splenomegaly (10 per cent).

Lymphadenopathy (50 per cent).

Nodules resembling those of rheumatoid arthritis (5 per cent).
Raynaud's phenomenon (30 per cent).

Fever (90 per cent) and *weight loss* (50 per cent).

Infections: Increased risk.

Gastro-intestinal: Non-specific symptoms common, loss of appetite, nausea, vomiting. Arteritis may cause ulceration, haemorrhage, necrosis and gangrene, or perforation. Rarely peritonitis, dysphagia (as in scleroderma), pancreatitis, or colitis.

Sjögren's Syndrome (25 per cent) usually asymptomatic.

REFERENCES

LABOWITZ, R., and SCHUMACHER, H. R. (1971), *Annals of Internal Medicine*, **74**, 911.
NOONAN, C. D., and others (1963), *Radiology*, **80**, 837.

PEKIN, T. J., and ZVAIFLER, N. J. (1970), *Arthritis and Rheumatism*, **13**, 777.
TAYLOR, R. T. (1970), *British Journal of Hospital Medicine*, **4**, 653.

TAKAYASU'S DISEASE (Aortic Arch Syndrome or Pulseless Disease)

A rare disease characterized by occlusion of major vessels, particularly those arising from the aortic arch. This is preceded by a systemic illness (pre-pulseless Takayasu's disease) with arthritis.

Incidence

F. 15 : 1.
Any age, but onset usually 15–40.
World-wide but commoner in Orient.
Arthritis or arthralgia occurs in about 50 per cent in the 'pre-pulseless' stage; pulse abnormalities appear 1–13 years later.

Joints affected

Usually neck or upper limbs (shoulders, elbows, wrists, and fingers).
Occasionally knees (30 per cent).
Rarely hips, ankles, or temporomandibular joints.
Polyarticular: occasionally migratory resembling rheumatic fever.

Symptoms

Joint and muscle pains.

Signs

Sometimes none; sometimes swelling or tenderness.

Course

Chronic with remissions and relapses, or episodic.
No joint residua.
Arterial complications may prove fatal.

Associations

1. Early pre-pulseless stage: Raynaud's phenomenon, rashes including erythema nodosum, pericarditis, iritis, episcleritis, arterial bruits, or tenderness.
2. Later loss of pulses and vascular insufficiency syndromes particularly transient cerebral ischaemic episodes, strokes, blindness, hypertension (renal artery stenosis), angina, myocardial infarction, heart failure, intestinal angina, haematemesis, melaena, claudication, and peripheral gangrene.

XR

Joints normal; aortography shows narrowing of affected vessels.

Laboratory

Raised E.S.R. in active stage.
Hyperglobulinaemia.
Latex test, L.E. cells and A.N.F. occasionally positive.

Treatment

1. Steroids suppress manifestations in the pre-pulseless stage including arthritis but have no effect on arterial changes.
2. Consider long-term anticoagulants.
3. Arterial surgery if necessary.

REFERENCES

STRACHAN, R. W. (1966), *Postgraduate Medical Journal*, 42, 464.

STRACHAN, R. W., and others (1966), *American Journal of Medicine*, 40, 560.

TEMPOROMANDIBULAR ARTHROPATHY

A condition of the older age-groups which differs from osteoarthritis in its sex incidence, transience, and histological and radiological features and is therefore described separately. It must be distinguished from the pain-dysfunction syndrome and other conditions affecting the temporomandibular joint which are described on p. 136. The pain-dysfunction syndrome affects younger patients and there are no radiological changes.

Incidence
F. 6 : 1.
Peak age 30–65.
40 per cent have a past history of pain-dysfunction syndrome—past trauma or fracture unusual.

Joints affected
Temporomandibular joint. Symptoms usually confined to one side but in 10 per cent the other side has been or will be involved.

Symptoms
Sudden or gradual onset of pain on jaw movement, worse towards evening. Crepitus and limitation of jaw movement common. Occasionally there is aching in the jaw or face.

Signs
Tenderness in 50 per cent, particularly with jaw open. Limitation of movement. Dental abnormalities unimportant.

Course
Severe discomfort usually persists for about 9 months, thereafter decreasing. Pain disappears in 50 per cent of cases within 1 year, in 75 per cent within 2 years, and in most cases within 5 years. Ankylosis does not occur.

XR
1. Irregular loss of bone density in the margin of the condyle adjacent to the joint, producing an irregular 'woolly' appearance.
2. Shallow saucer-shaped erosion of the condyle.
3. Osteophytes occasionally (20 per cent). Tomography or transpharyngeal projection useful to visualize the joint.
After a few years the condyle is remineralized and remodelled with alteration in shape and reduction in size of the condyle.

Laboratory
Unhelpful. Normal E.S.R.

Treatment
1. Relief of pain. Simple analgesics; heat and massage.
2. Correction of malocclusion and other dental abnormalities.
3. Intra-articular hydrocortisone in resistant cases—0·5 ml. (12·5 mg. of prednisolone).
4. Condylectomy as a last resort.

REFERENCES

TOLLER, P. A. (1973), *British Dental Journal*, **134**, 773.   TOLLER, P. A. (1974), *Proceedings of the Royal Society of Medicine*, **67**, 153.

TEMPOROMANDIBULAR JOINT DISORDERS

The following conditions affect the temporomandibular joint:

1. The pain-dysfunction syndrome, described below. This resembles in some respects the syndrome described by Costen which is not now regarded as an entity.

2. Temporomandibular arthropathy; see p. 135.

3. Rheumatoid arthritis. The temporomandibular joint is affected in 50 per cent of cases at some time during the course of the disease. The disorder, characterized by pain, stiffness, local tenderness, crepitus, and limitation of jaw opening with erosions on X-ray, usually lasts for a few months and seldom recurs. Treatment with analgesic and anti-inflammatory drugs relieves pain and local steroid injection is not usually necessary.

4. Ankylosing spondylitis rarely affects the temporomandibular joint but once involved, the condition is progressive and may result in severe restriction of jaw opening and ankylosis. Condylectomy or arthroplasty is then required.

5. Still's disease is also a rare cause of temporomandibular arthritis but there are two important consequences. Premature closure of the epiphysis may lead to micrognathia and ankylosis may occur.

6. Other arthropathies rarely affect the joint. Traumatic arthritis may follow a blow or dental treatment. Septic or tuberculous arthritis may arise either from spread in the blood-stream or from ears, mastoid, teeth, or parotids. Pain in the joint may be the consequence of fracture or tumours of the condyle.

Incidence
F. 5 : 1.
Peak age 20–50.
Often anxious bruxists (teeth grinders) with emotional problems.

Joints affected
Temporomandibular joint; usually unilateral.

Symptoms
1. Dull, diffuse, constant pain in the region of the joint or in the ear or face, rarely radiating to the neck and shoulder, aggravated by chewing, worst in the morning, when the jaw may also be stiff.
2. Limitation of jaw movement, 'clicking' or grating on chewing, and rarely 'locking', subluxation or dislocation.
   Sudden onset of symptoms may follow yawning, prolonged dental treatment, or changes in occlusion, e.g., after dental extraction.

Signs
Painful limitation of movement; tenderness over the joint and muscles of mastication. Sometimes evidence of malocclusion; the upper incisor teeth may overlap the lower.

Course
Most cases recover within 1 year but there may be residual limitation of jaw movement.

XR
Normal.

Laboratory
Unhelpful.

Treatment
1. Relief of pain. Simple analgesics; injection of the joint or muscles with local anaesthetic; heat and massage. Tranquillizers may help.
2. Correction of malocclusion by dental therapy.
3. Exercises.

REFERENCE

SCHWARTZ, L., and CHAYES, C. M. (1968), *Facial Pain and Mandibular Dysfunction.* Philadelphia: Saunders.

TENNIS ELBOW

A common traumatic condition arising at the origin of the extensor muscles of the forearm from the lateral humeral epicondyle. It occurs in adults of either sex and is caused by repeated forceful movements of the elbow including tennis but more often housework or manual occupations. There is pain in the elbow, usually unilateral and more commonly in the dominant limb, aggravated by use. Examination in most cases reveals only tenderness over the lateral humeral epicondyle; rarely there is local swelling, warmth, and erythema but the joint is otherwise normal. XR is normal. Injection of hydrocortisone into the tender area is usually curative but relapse may occur especially if the precipitating injury is repeated. Golfer's elbow is a similar but less common condition of the origin of the flexor muscles of the forearm from the medial humeral epicondyle.

TENNIS LEG

Caused by a traumatic tear at the musculotendinous junction of the medial belly of the gastrocnemius muscle. It produces a sudden sharp pain which makes the player believe he has been struck from behind. Palpation reveals a gap in the muscle. Like tennis elbow and tennis thumb, it is not confined to tennis players and the most famous case was that of Dr. W. G. Grace who sustained such an injury after making 60 runs at Lords on 12 June 1884. He was successfully treated by elevation of the leg and firm strapping and completed his innings on the following day. Similar symptoms may be produced by rupture of the Achilles tendon which may require surgery.

REFERENCE

British Medical Journal (1969), **1**, 115.

TENNIS THUMB

A variety of acute calcific periarthritis, affecting the insertion of the flexor pollicis longus tendon into the distal phalanx of the thumb. There is acute pain and XR shows calcification.

REFERENCE

OLDFIELD, M. C. (1951), *Lancet*, **1**, 1151.

THIEMANN'S DISEASE

A rare familial condition characterized by avascular necrosis of the epiphyses of the small joints of the hands or feet. Because it occurs in childhood and adolescence, it may be mistaken for juvenile chronic arthritis or rheumatoid arthritis.

Incidence
Very rare.
Autosomal dominant—good penetrance.
Onset age 4–40, usually in childhood, immediately before puberty.

Joints affected
P.I.P. joints of 2nd, 3rd and 4th fingers (3rd commonest). Occasionally other I.P. joints of hand, I.P. joints of great toe, P.I.P. joints of toes, or M.C.P. or M.T.P. joints. Bilateral and symmetrical.

Symptoms
Progressive enlargement of P.I.P. joints. Sometimes pain and stiffness.

Signs
Affected joints are swollen and tender but not red or warm. Restriction of movement. Later flexion deformities. First phalanges are short.

Course
Usually mild with minor discomfort and function preserved.

Associations
None.

Laboratory
No diagnostic tests.
Normal E.S.R.
Negative latex tests.

137

THIEMANN'S DISEASE (*continued*)

XR
Irregularity, flattening, fragmentation and
beaking of epiphysis. Epiphysis may disappear. Irregularity and cupping of the base
of the second phalanx.

Treatment
Not required.

REFERENCE

RUBINSTEIN, H. M. (1975), *Arthritis and Rheumatism,* **18,** 357.

THYROID ACROPACHY

A rare disorder, characterized by swelling of the soft tissues of the extremities associated with
clubbing, exophthalmos, and pretibial myxoedema. It follows successful treatment of
hyperthyroidism.

Incidence
M. = F.
Adults—any age.
1 per cent of cases of hyperthyroidism.
Occurs 2–20 years after onset of hyper-
thyroidism.

Joints affected
Affects soft tissues of fingers and toes.
Bilateral and symmetrical.

Symptoms
Painless soft-tissue swelling of fingers and
toes.
Stiffness common.

Signs
Soft-tissue swelling.
No warmth or tenderness.

Course
Continues unchanged for years, occasionally
with eventual complete or partial remission.

Associations
1. Past history of hyperthyroidism,
   exophthalmos (100 per cent), and
   pretibial myxoedema (80 per cent) usually
   in that order.
2. 50 per cent are hypothyroid at onset of
   acropachy; 40 per cent euthyroid; 10 per
   cent hyperthyroid.
3. Clubbing (90 per cent).

XR
'Bubbly' irregular periosteal new bone
formation involving shafts of metacarpals,
metatarsals, and phalanges.

Laboratory
Unhelpful.
E.S.R. normal.

Treatment
Correct thyroid status but this has no effect
on acropachy.
No specific treatment required.

REFERENCE

GIMLETTE, T. M. D. (1960), *Lancet,* **1,** 22.

TIETZE'S SYNDROME

A rare non-hereditary condition, characterized by attacks of painful swelling of a costal cartilage. Its importance lies in the differential diagnosis of angina and intrathoracic malignancy.

Incidence
M. = F.
Any age; peak 20–40.

Joints affected
Second (45 per cent) and third (20 per cent) costosternal junctions commonest; occasionally first or fourth (15 per cent); rarely other costosternal junctions or sternoclavicular joints.
One site only in 80 per cent; where multiple sites are involved, 80 per cent are unilateral.

Symptoms
Upper anterior chest pain and swelling; onset sudden or gradual. Pain is aggravated by coughing and sneezing.

Signs
Tender swelling of costal cartilage.

Course
Attacks usually last only a few hours or days, but recur at irregular intervals. The condition usually subsides completely within a few months, but rarely lasts up to 10 years.

Associations
No systemic manifestations.
Exclude other causes of chest pain particularly malignancy, also ankylosing spondylitis which causes similar symptoms.

XR
Normal.
Calcification of costal cartilages is common, but of little significance.

Laboratory
Unhelpful.
E.S.R. normal.

Treatment
1. Aspirin and other anti-inflammatory drugs.
2. Local heat.
3. Local injection of anaesthetic and hydrocortisone.

REFERENCE

LEVEY, G. S., and CALABRO, J. J. (1962), *Arthritis and Rheumatism*, 5, 261.

TRANSIENT OSTEOPOROSIS OF THE HIP

A rare condition in which painful limitation of movement of the hip is associated with radiological osteoporosis. It recovers completely, but is important in the differential diagnosis of tuberculosis.

Incidence
Physically active males.
Age 30–60.

Joints affected
Hip.
Unilateral; monarticular.

Symptoms
Pain in the hip or knee, worse on weight bearing.
Limp.
Sudden onset in 50 per cent.

Signs
Painful limitation of movement.
Local tenderness.

Course
Complete recovery within 6 months. 30 per cent have an episode involving the opposite hip months or years later.

XR
Osteoporosis limited to the femoral head, either generalized or 'mottled'. Changes may not appear for 4–6 weeks after onset of symptoms.
CXR for tuberculosis.

Laboratory
Normal E.S.R.
If in doubt, exploration and biopsy to exclude tuberculosis.

Treatment
1. Analgesics.
2. Walking stick may help. Immobilization is not necessary.

REFERENCE

LEQUESNE, M. (1968), *Annals of the Rheumatic Diseases*, **27**, 463.

TRANSIENT PAINFUL OSTEOPOROSIS

A rare condition of unknown aetiology in which episodes of pain in and around the joints of the lower limb are accompanied by radiological and histological evidence of osteoporosis. The condition resembles Sudeck's post-traumatic atrophy (*see* p. 127) but the severe burning, throbbing pain, muscle spasm, skin changes and restriction of passive joint movement do not occur.

Incidence
Age 40–60.
F. 2 : 1.

Joints affected
Ankle and foot usually involved at some time. Occasionally knee, hip or big toe.
Usually one joint at a time unless attacks overlap.

Symptoms
Gradual onset of joint pain, becoming very severe and spreading to involve surrounding areas, aggravated by weight-bearing.
Difficulty in walking—stick or crutch often required because of the severity of the pain.
No morning stiffness.

Signs
Limitation of active but not passive joint movement. Tenderness of adjacent bones.
Joints may be otherwise normal. If ankle is involved, diffuse swelling spreading to the foot is characteristic.
Warmth and erythema unusual and slight.
Occasionally knee effusion.

Course
Pain increases over weeks or months, remains very severe for a few months, then subsides, disappearing usually completely within 6–12 months. Occasionally pain lasts longer or slight pain remains after the attack.
Recurrence is common—up to 12 episodes reported.

Associations
No preceding trauma or other disease.

TRANSIENT PAINFUL OSTEOPOROSIS (*continued*)

XR

Diminished bone density around the affected joint, diffuse at first but later patchy, returning to normal with resolution which may take years. May be followed by coarse irregular trabecular pattern.
No erosions (cf. tuberculosis).

Laboratory

E.S.R. usually normal—occasionally slightly increased.
Bone biopsy: osteoporosis.

Treatment

1. Reassurance.
2. Analgesics.
3. Maintain mobility as far as possible during the acute stage with the aid of sticks, etc.
4. Physiotherapy as recovery proceeds.
5. In the difficult case steroids are worth trying (prednisolone 40 mg. daily at first, reducing over a few months).

REFERENCE

LANGLOH, N. D., and others (1973), *Journal of Bone and Joint Surgery*, **55A**, 1188.

TRANSIENT SYNOVITIS OF THE HIP (Irritable or Observation Hip)

A benign condition of the hip in children, characterized by an episode of painful limitation of movement. Its importance lies in the differential diagnosis of septic or tuberculous infection and Perthes' disease.

Incidence

M. 3 : 2.
Children 2–15, peak 5–10.
Rare in adults.

Joints affected

Hip.
Unilateral; monarticular.

Symptoms

Sudden onset of pain, radiating to thigh or knee, causing limp.

Signs

Limitation of movement; hip may be held in flexion and adduction.
Slight fever occasionally.

Course

Persists for weeks or rarely months, but eventually resolves completely.
Rarely leads to early osteoarthritis.

XR

Normal.

Laboratory

E.S.R. usually normal.
W.B.C. normal.
Synovial fluid: sterile.
Biopsy: non-specific synovitis.

Treatment

Rest.
Analgesics.

REFERENCE

British Medical Journal (1969), **1**, 333.

ACUTE TRAUMATIC ARTHRITIS

Arthritis due to direct or indirect injury. This usually affects normal joints, but may aggravate existing joint disease such as osteoarthritis or meniscus injuries and other mechanical derangements.

Incidence

Peak in young adult males.

Joints affected

Depends upon the nature of the injury.
Knee commonest.
Often ankle or wrist.
Monarticular.

Symptoms

Sudden onset of pain and swelling.
History of trauma is usual but is often obtainable in any type of acute arthritis.

Signs

Joint is warm and swollen with effusion and painful limitation of movement.

Course

Spontaneous recovery within 6 weeks.
Only if trauma is repeated does osteoarthritis develop later.

XR

Normal.
Exclude associated fracture.

Laboratory

E.S.R. and other tests normal.
Synovial fluid: viscous. Little or no increase in cells. May be blood-stained.

Treatment

1. Rest in acute stage. Strapping and splintage may be helpful.
2. Analgesic and anti-inflammatory drugs.
3. Joint aspiration is hazardous and unnecessary in most cases. It may speed recovery after haemarthrosis if there is a large, tense effusion.
4. Intra-articular steroids are best avoided especially in sportsmen who suffer repeated trauma. One injection only may be given in a case which is failing to respond to other measures.
5. Physiotherapy after the acute stage to maintain mobility and restore muscle power.

TRAVELLER'S ANKLE

Ankle swelling and discomfort often follows long journeys by bus or aeroplane and is probably due to venous stasis. It does not occur in the drivers of cars except in the left leg of drivers of automatic cars and can be avoided by regular movement.

REFERENCE

JOHNSON, H. D. (1973), *British Medical Journal*, 3, 109.

TROCHANTERIC SYNDROME

A soft-tissue syndrome similar to those which occur in the shoulder (*see* Frozen Shoulder). It arises in the abductor mechanism of the hip and soft-tissue calcification is seen on XR in about one-third of cases. There is pain and tenderness in the region of the greater trochanter, radiating down the posterolateral thigh and therefore mistaken on occasions for sciatica. Onset is typically sudden. Treatment: Local injection of prednisolone.

REFERENCE

LEONARD, M. H. (1958), *Journal of the American Medical Association*, **168**, 175.

TUBERCULOUS ARTHRITIS or SPONDYLITIS

Infection of joint or spine with *Mycobacterium tuberculosis*. The condition is now rare in Great Britain.

Incidence

M. > F.

Any age; commoner in children and elderly, debilitated and malnourished.

Joints affected

Spine, particularly dorsal (40 per cent) and hip (25 per cent) commonest.
Also knee (15 per cent), ankle or foot (5 per cent), sacro-iliac joint (5 per cent).
Rarely shoulder, elbow, wrist, or pubis.
Hip involvement is commoner in children (40 per cent).
Usually monarticular.

Symptoms

Insidious onset with swelling and restricted movement.
Pain slight at first and often worse at end of day.
Muscle spasms occur at night ('night starts' in children).
Limp common if hip involved.
Spinal involvement: back, root, or girdle pain; paraplegia; angular kyphosis.

Signs

Early: none.
Later joint is swollen, warm, and slightly tender with limitation of all movements due to muscle spasm. Muscle wasting around affected joint. Flexion deformity common. Skin over superficial lesions may be cold and bluish-red.

Course

Untreated progresses rapidly to deformity and joint destruction.
Spinal involvement carries risk of paraplegia. Other complications are formation of cold abscess or sinus.

Associations

1. Other tuberculous foci present in 50 per cent, pulmonary T.B. commonest. Look for lymphadenopathy.
2. Tenosynovitis (rare).

XR

Joints:
1. Early: normal or osteoporosis.
2. Later diminished joint space.
3. Erosions and rarely subarticular cysts with sclerotic margins.
4. Smudgy irregular bone outline from destructive changes.

Spine:
1. Narrowing of disc space.
2. Areas of osteoporosis and later destructive changes in adjacent vertebrae.

Laboratory

Bacteriological confirmation by direct examination, culture and guinea-pig inoculation of synovial fluid or biopsy material.
Characteristic histological changes on biopsy.
Synovial fluid: turbid with high mononuclear cell count.
E.S.R.: raised.
Blood-count variable, often normal; relative lymphocytosis characteristic.
Mantoux test: strongly positive supports the diagnosis especially in children (inquire for past B.C.G. vaccination). Tuberculosis unlikely with negative Mantoux.

Treatment

Chemotherapy (streptomycin, rifampicin, and isoniazid until sensitivity available).
Continue for 2 years.
Check streptomycin blood level.
Joints:
1. Rest in acute stage, but with daily passive movements to maintain mobility.
2. Traction or splinting to correct or prevent deformity.
3. Indications for surgical débridement (preferably after at least 3 weeks of chemotherapy).
   a. Abscess formation.
   b. Presence of grossly diseased bone, sequestra, or other debris.
   c. Delayed recovery.
Spine: 3 weeks' immobilization in a plaster bed, plus chemotherapy, then surgical débridement and fusion.

REFERENCE

SOMERVILLE, E. W., and WILKINSON, M. C. (1965), *Girdlestone's Tuberculosis of Bone and Joint*, 3rd ed. London: Oxford University Press.

TUMORAL CALCINOSIS

A rare condition of unknown aetiology affecting predominantly coloured races (M. = F., any age) which presents with painless joint swelling: there is a slowly growing subcutaneous tumour, most commonly adjacent to the hip or elbow, sometimes shoulder, knee, wrist, or other joints. The tumours are usually single. Rarely there is a discharge of chalky fluid. XR confirms calcification. Histology is characteristic and excision cures.

REFERENCE

SLAVIN, G., and others (1973), *British Medical Journal*, 1, 147.

TYPHOID FEVER

A serious febrile illness due to infection with *Salmonella typhi*. Arthritis is of the following types:

1. *Arthralgia* is common in the early stages, and is a presenting symptom of typhoid in about 50 per cent of patients.
2. *Salmonella arthritis* (*see* p. 118)
   and
3. *Post-salmonella arthritis* (*see* p. 103) are rare complications, affecting 1 per cent of patients or less.
4. *Typhoid spine* is a low-grade osteomyelitis of the spine which appears months or years after an attack of typhoid fever. With the advent of antibiotic therapy the condition has become exceptionally rare.

Treatment: Chloramphenicol.

REFERENCE

HUCKSTEP, R. L. (1962), *Typhoid Fever*. Edinburgh: Livingstone.

URTICARIA

Attacks of urticaria are often accompanied by arthralgia, painful joints being associated with overlying skin lesions and lasting for a few hours. Bouts of polyarthralgia associated with fever and urticaria are also a feature of a rare syndrome inherited as an autosomal dominant, associated with deafness and amyloidosis.

REFERENCE

MUCKLE, T. J., and WELLS, M. (1962), *Quarterly Journal of Medicine*, 31, 235.

VACCINATION

Monarticular arthritis resembling septic arthritis has been described after small-pox vaccination. Joint fluid was purulent with a neutrophil leucocytosis and vaccinia virus was cultured from it. A transient polyarthritis sometimes follows rubella vaccination (*see* p. 117). Arthralgia may occur with febrile reactions to other vaccines, e.g., TAB.

REFERENCE

SILBY, H. M., and others (1965), *Annals of Internal Medicine*, 62, 347.

VARICELLA (Chicken-pox)

Arthritis is not usually a complication of varicella infection but a case has been reported with transient arthritis of one knee, starting on the day after the appearance of the rash. The joint was painful and swollen with marked limitation of movement and effusion. Synovial fluid was inflammatory with a predominantly mononuclear leucocytosis; the virus was not recovered from the fluid.

REFERENCE

WARD, J. R., and BISHOP, B. (1970), *Journal of the American Medical Association*, **212**, 1954.

VIRAL HEPATITIS

Type-A (short incubation period) or type-B (long incubation period, serum hepatitis) virus hepatitis typically manifest as an attack of jaundice, preceded by constitutional features such as malaise, fever, anorexia, and sometimes arthritis. Cases with arthritis tend to have low complement levels and circulating hepatitis-associated (Australia) antigen suggesting the presence of circulating antigen–antibody complexes.

Incidence

M. = F.
Young adults.
10 per cent have joint pains; commoner with type-B virus infection.
Occurs at prodromal stage preceding jaundice.

Joints affected

P.I.P. joints of hands common.
Occasionally knees, shoulders, hips, elbows, ankles, and spine.
Bilateral and symmetrical.

Symptoms

Sudden onset of joint pain and stiffness.
Morning stiffness often severe.
Malaise and anorexia.
Inquire for drug addiction and recent blood transfusion.

Signs

None (50 per cent) or red, warm, tender joints.
Small effusion rarely present.
Fever sometimes.

Course

Arthritis recovers completely within 3 weeks, usually when jaundice appears.

Associations

1. Urticaria (common) and angioneurotic oedema (rare).
2. Subsequent jaundice.

XR

Normal.

Laboratory

Raised transaminases and later bilirubin.
E.S.R. slightly raised.
Latex test or A.N.F. rarely positive.
Check complement level and hepatitis-associated antigen.
Synovial fluid: inflammatory; W.B.C. up to $20,000 \times 10^9/\text{dl.}$, mainly mononulcears.
Low complement level.

Treatment

Analgesics.

REFERENCES

ALPERT, E., and others (1971), *New England Journal of Medicine*, **285**, 185.

ONION, D. K., and others (1971), *Annals of Internal Medicine*, **75**, 29.

WEGENER'S GRANULOMATOSIS

A rare condition in which an invasive necrotizing granulomatous lesion of the nose is associated with a systemic arteritic illness resembling polyarteritis nodosa.

Incidence

M. 2 : 1.
Any age, peak 25–55.
Arthritis in 30 per cent, during the course of the disease.

Joints affected

Polyarticular.
Affects large or small joints.
Often migratory.

Symptoms

Joint pain and swelling.

Signs

Joints are often warm, red, and swollen.
Effusion may be present.
Fever usually present intermittently.

Course

Arthritis is usually episodic and resolves without residua.
The disease is usually fatal within a year or two.
Prolonged remission may be induced by azathioprine.

Associations

1. Nasal congestion with blood-stained discharge leading to nasal obstruction and ulceration of surrounding cartilage and bone.
2. Renal disease; albuminuria with red and white cells in the urine, progressing to renal failure.
3. Pulmonary changes secondary to nasal disease: cough, haemoptysis, pneumonia.
4. Other systemic manifestations of polyarteritis nodosa occasionally.

XR

Normal.

Laboratory

Anaemia, leucocytosis, and raised E.S.R.
Diagnosis confirmed by biopsy of nasal granuloma.

Treatment

1. Azathioprine.
2. Steroids may control systemic manifestations including arthritis.

Variants

Direct invasion of the temporomandibular joint may occur in the late stage.

REFERENCE

ALDO, M. A., and others (1970), *Archives of Internal Medicine*, **126**, 298.

FAHEY, J. L., and others (1954), *American Journal of Medicine*, **17**, 168.

WEIL'S DISEASE (Leptospirosis)

Infection with the spirochaete, *Leptospira icterohaemorrhagiae*, acquired from water contaminated by rats or other rodents, and found particularly in sewer workers. There is a sudden onset of fever, headache, myalgia, and, on about the fourth day, jaundice: widespread haemorrhages may occur. Arthritis is very rare, but has been reported, affecting the hip and spine. The diagnosis may be confirmed by examination of a blood-film, blood-culture, and agglutination test. Treatment: Penicillin.

REFERENCE

JACOBS, J. H. (1951), *Annals of the Rheumatic Diseases*, **10**, 61.

WERNER'S SYNDROME (Adult Progeria)

A rare disorder inherited as an autosomal recessive character, particularly affecting Jews and characterized by premature senility and corresponding changes in various structures including joints. A similar arthritis occurs in *progeria* (Hutchinson–Gilford syndrome), a very rare non-hereditary condition starting in the first 3 years of life, with similar clinical features, but no cataracts.

Incidence

M. = F.
Onset age 15–40.
Arthritis is common.

Joints affected

Hands, feet, ankles, and spine, common.
Distal interphalangeal joints affected most severely.
Often knees and elbows; occasionally shoulders and hips.

Symptoms

Pain.
Deformities.

Signs

Bony swelling.
Tenderness.
Limitation of movement.
Ulnar deviation of hands and bizarre deformities of toes may resemble rheumatoid arthritis.

Course

Chronic, progressing slowly to severe deformities particularly of hands and feet. Early death from vascular disease or malignancy.

Associations

1. Features of premature ageing: baldness, grey hair, weak high-pitched voice.
2. Cataracts.
3. Arteriosclerosis causing angina, myocardial infarction, and peripheral vascular disease.
4. Loss of subcutaneous fat; atrophy of skin. Tight atrophic skin over fingers resembles scleroderma. Ulcers may occur around ankles.
5. Typical appearance: short stature, beak nose, wasting.
6. Hypogonadism; diabetes mellitus in 20 per cent.
7. Malignant tumours.

XR

1. Degenerative changes in joints: loss of joint space, sclerosis, osteophytes, cysts. Bone destruction may be seen in the toes, resembling neuropathic changes.
2. Generalized osteoporosis.
3. Calcification of arteries and soft tissues.

Laboratory

No specific histological or biochemical features.

Treatment

Symptomatic.

REFERENCES

GRANT, A. P. (1957), *Ulster Medical Journal*, 26, 65.
JACOBSON, H. G., and others (1960), *Radiology*, 74, 373.

THANNHAUSER, S. J. (1945), *Annals of Internal Medicine*, 23, 559.

WHIPPLE'S DISEASE

A rare disease in which the small intestine and lymph-nodes are infiltrated with masses of macrophages containing material which stains with periodic-acid-Schiff reagent. There is a clinical triad of steatorrhoea, lymphadenopathy, and arthritis. It is rarely associated with spinal and sacro-iliac changes of ankylosing spondylitis.

Incidence

M. 4 : 1.
Age 30–60.
60 per cent have arthritis.
Arthritis usually precedes gastro-intestinal features, sometimes by many years.

Joints affected

Knees, ankles, shoulders, and wrists commonly. Spine, P.I.P. and M.C.P. joints, elbows, and feet occasionally.
One or many joints.
Sometimes migratory and mistaken for rheumatic fever.

Symptoms

Pain (often slight).
Stiffness and swelling.

Signs

Affected joints usually swollen and tender with limitation of movement and effusion; occasionally hot and red.

Course

Attacks last a few days or weeks and resolve spontaneously, recurring at irregular intervals of months or years.
Deformity seldom occurs.

Associations

1. Abdominal pain, diarrhoea, and weight-loss.
2. Pigmentation (65 per cent) may suggest Addison's disease.
3. Peripheral lymphadenopathy (50 per cent).
4. Purpura (30 per cent).

XR

Normal.

Laboratory

Raised E.S.R.
Latex test negative.
Steatorrhoea: raised faecal fat, etc.
Biopsies of small bowel and lymph-node confirm the diagnosis.

Treatment

1. Tetracycline.
2. Analgesic and anti-inflammatory drugs.

REFERENCES

CAUGHEY, D. E., and BYWATERS, E. G. L. (1963), Annals of the Rheumatic Diseases, **22**, 327.
FARNAN, P. (1959), Quarterly Journal of Medicine, **28**, 163.

WHIPPLE, G. H. (1907), Bulletin of the Johns Hopkins Hospital, **18**, 382.

WILSON'S DISEASE

A rare disorder, inherited as an autosomal recessive, characterized by accumulation of copper in tissues such as brain, liver, and kidney. A degenerative arthropathy resembling osteoarthritis (described below) is common in adults. Joint pain is rarely due to rickets[3] (*see* p. 92) or penicillamine therapy which may cause arthralgia or a lupus-like syndrome.[4]

Incidence

M. = F.
Age at onset 5–40, peak 10–15.
Arthritis begins at about age 30.
Radiological skeletal abnormalities found in 70 per cent of cases.

Joints affected

Hands, wrists, and knees commonest.
Sometimes elbows, shoulders, and hips.
Bilateral and symmetrical.

Symptoms

Joint pain.
Later limitation of motion.
No morning stiffness.

Signs

Bony swelling, tenderness, and crepitus.
No warmth or erythema.

Course

Resembles osteoarthritis.
Severe cases progress to incapacity within a a few years.

Associations

1. Cirrhosis of the liver, jaundice, malaise, and abdominal pain.
2. Neuropsychiatric disease; insidious deterioration of intellect followed by tremor, cogwheel rigidity, ataxia, and choreiform movements.
3. Kayser-Fleischer ring (greenish-brown ring around the cornea). If in doubt, examine under slit lamp.

XR

1. Fragmentation of bone at joint margins causing loose bodies.
2. Degenerative changes with loss of joint space, sclerosis, and osteophytes.
3. Thin bones; pseudofractures; true fractures.
4. Minor degree of chondrocalcinosis.

Laboratory

1. 24-hour urine copper raised.
2. Serum copper and caeruloplasmin (oxidase activity) reduced.
3. If in doubt, liver biopsy and quantitative copper estimation, or radioactive copper test, or effect of penicillamine on urinary copper.
4. Synovial fluid: non-inflammatory.
5. Synovial biopsy: no excess of copper demonstrable.

Treatment

D-penicillamine.
Analgesics as required.

REFERENCES

[1] FELLER, E. R., and SCHUMACHER, H. R. (1972), *Arthritis and Rheumatism,* **15,** 259.
[2] FINBY, N., and BEARN, A. G. (1958), *American Journal of Roentgenology,* **79,** 603.
[3] CAVALLINO, R., and GROSSMAN, H. (1968), *Radiology,* **90,** 493.
[4] HARPEY, J. P., and others (1971), *Lancet,* **1,** 292.

WINCHESTER SYNDROME (Acid Mucopolysaccharidosis)

A very rare inherited mucopolysaccharide storage disease characterized by intracellular accumulation of uronic acid. It may be mistaken for juvenile chronic arthritis.

Incidence
Very rare.
Autosomal recessive inheritance.
Onset within the first two years of life.

Joints affected
Polyarticular. Large and small joints.
Bilateral and symmetrical.
Spine also affected.

Clinical Features
Painful swollen joints—not red or warm.
Restriction of movement.

Course
Progresses to severe joint contractures, grotesque deformities, ankylosis and great disability.

Associated Features
1. Corneal opacities.
2. Coarse facial features with thick lips, fleshy nose and prominant forehead.
3. Retarded growth.
4. ECG changes compatible with cardio-myopathy.
MENTALLY NORMAL.
No hepatosplenomegaly.

XR
Changes best seen in wrists, hands and knees.
1. Osteoporosis.
2. Narrowing of shafts of long bones with widening (flaring) of metaphysis.
3. Irregularity and progressive destructive changes in epiphyses and ends of long bones.
   Leads to disappearance of carpal bones and 'whittling' of ends of metacarpals.
4. May progress to ankylosis of joints.
5. Atlanto-axial subluxation may occur.
6. Delayed closure of fontanelles and tooth eruption.

Laboratory
Unhelpful.
No urinary mucopolysaccharides.

Treatment
Symptomatic. Try to preserve mobility.
Rehabilitation.

REFERENCE

WINCHESTER, P., and others (1969), *American Journal of Roentgenology*, **106**, 121.

XIPHOID SYNDROME

A rare benign syndrome, often due to trauma, characterized by pain in the xiphisternum. The condition is important only because of its differentiation from other causes of pain localized to the anterior chest wall.

1. Cardiac, pleural, oesophageal, and gastric lesions.
2. Soft-tissue syndromes:
   a. *Tietze's disease (see* p. 139).
   b. *Tumours,* e.g., rib secondaries or multiple myeloma.
   c. *Rib fracture.*
   d. *Asher's precordial catch.*
   e. *Herpes zoster.*
   f. *Ankylosing spondylitis.*
   g. *Spinal root compression.*
   h. *Relapsing polychondritis (see* p. 111).

Incidence
M. = F.
Adults only.

Joints affected
Xiphisternum.

Symptoms
Pains centring around and emanating from the xiphisternum, which may radiate to the precordium, epigastrium, shoulder or back, aggravated by pressure, abdominal distension, lifting, stooping, bending, or twisting.
May follow local injury such as a blow to the area.

Signs
Tender xiphoid process, which may be either unduly prominent or may be mobile.

Course
Persists for weeks or months but disappears eventually.
Sometimes recurrent.

XR
Normal.

Laboratory
Unhelpful.

Treatment
Analgesics.
Reassurance ('heart trouble' often suspected by the patient).

REFERENCE

WEHRMACHER, W. H. (1958), *Medical Clinics of North America,* **42**, 111.

YAWS

A non-venereal treponemal infection caused by *Treponema pertenue*, found in tropical parts of Africa, South America, the Caribbean, and the Far East. Infection is acquired by direct contact with the skin lesions. A primary papillomatous lesion develops at the site of infection with secondary lesions elsewhere, particularly in the groins, perineum, and axillae. The disease is commonest in childhood. Periostitis and osteitis are common in the early or later stages of the disease and arthritis is a rare accompaniment. There is joint pain and swelling, usually mon-articular, and affecting large joints. XR shows well-defined areas of porosis or periosteal deposits adjacent to the affected joint. W.R. and T.P.I. are positive and the condition must be distinguished from syphilis on clinical grounds. Penicillin provides effective treatment.

REFERENCE

HACKETT, C. J. (1951), *Bone Lesions of Yaws in Uganda*. Oxford: Blackwell.

YERSINIA ARTHRITIS

Infection with *Yersinia* (*Pasteurella*) *enterocolitica*[1] or *pseudotuberculosis*[2] usually causes a mild gastro-intestinal illness with fever, abdominal pain, and diarrhoea or an acute appendicitis-like condition due to either mesenteric adenitis or terminal ileitis. The arthritis which may follow is probably not due to direct bacterial infection of the joint, but to a 'reaction' on the part of the host. *Y. enterocolitica* infection may also cause Reiter's syndrome (*see* p. 110).

Incidence

M. = F.
Age 15–40.
Arthritis usually follows diarrhoea or abdominal pain by up to 3 weeks—rarely precedes gastro-intestinal symptoms by up to 3 days.

Joints affected

Polyarticular.
Lower limb predominantly.
Knees (50 per cent), ankles (50 per cent), fingers, toes, and wrist commonest.
Occasionally hip, lumbar spine, sacro-iliac joint, shoulder, or temporomandibular joint.
Usually asymmetrical.

Symptoms

Acute onset of severe pain and swelling.

Signs

Joints are usually tender and swollen; often red and warm with effusion.
Fever common.

Course

Gastro-intestinal symptoms last up to 1 week.
Arthritis lasts up to 6 months, but resolves without deformities.

Associations

1. Diarrhoea and abdominal pain.
2. Muscular pain and stiffness.
3. Erythema nodosum occasionally.
4. Rare manifestations include unilateral conjunctivitis, pneumonitis, hilar lymphadenopathy, meningitis, lymph-adenopathy, and splenomegaly.

XR

Normal.

Laboratory

E.S.R. raised.
Often leucocytosis.
Positive agglutination test for *Yersinia*; rising titre.
False-positive agglutination test for *Brucella*.
Latex test negative.
Synovial fluid: inflammatory with W.B.C. up to $20,000 \times 10^9$/dl., predominantly polymorphs; sterile on culture.
HLA B27 in 60 per cent.

Treatment

Salicylates and other anti-inflammatory drugs.
Antibiotics have no effect.

REFERENCES

[1] AHVONEN, P., and others (1969), *Acta Rheumatologica Scandinavica*, **15**, 232

[2] HÄLLSTRÖM, K., and others (1972), *Acta Medical Scandinavica*, **191**, 485.

INDEX

Figures in bold type indicate main references

153